ANNUAL REVIEW OF NURSING RESEARCH

Volume 8, 1990

ANNUAL REVIEW OF NURSING RESEARCH

Volume 8

Joyce J. Fitzpatrick, Ph.D.
Roma Lee Taunton, Ph.D.
Jeanne Quint Benoliel, D.N.Sc.

Editors

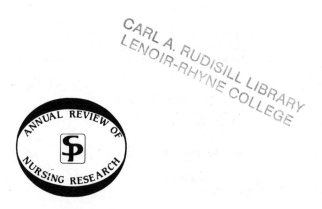

SPRINGER PUBLISHING COMPANY
New York

Order ANNUAL REVIEW OF NURSING RESEARCH, Volume 9, 1991,
prior to publication and receive a 10% discount. An order coupon can be
found at the back of this volume.

Springer Publishing Company, Inc.
536 Broadway
New York, NY 10012

90 91 92 93 94 / 5 4 3 2 1

ISBN-0-8261-4357-1
ISSN-0739-6686

ANNUAL REVIEW OF NURSING RESEARCH is indexed in *Cumulative
Index to Nursing and Allied Health Literature and Index Medicus.*

Printed in the United States of America

Contents

Preface

The *Annual Review of Nursing Research* series has been a welcome addition to the scientific literature in nursing. In their review and analysis of the literature, authors have contributed to the development of nursing knowledge for the discipline. They also have continued to project future research directions. These critical reviews and future projections set the stage for continued discipline growth.

Research reviewed for Volume 8 follows the established format for five major parts: Nursing Practice, Nursing Care Delivery, Nursing Education, the Profession of Nursing, and Other Research. Authors are selected based on their scientific expertise in an identified area.

The chapters under Nursing Practice for the present volume are focused on physiological dimensions of nursing; this also was the case for Volume 7. Marie J. Cowan reviews cardiovascular nursing research; Carolyn E. Carlson and Rosemarie B. King review research on prevention of pressure sores; Elizabeth M. Burns examines stress during the brain growth spurt; and Kathleen A. O'Connell reviews research on smoking and relapse. Chapters in this area in Volumes 1 and 4 were focused on human development along the life span, chapters in Volume 2 on family, and Volume 3 on community, Volume 5 on human responses to actual and potential health problems, chapters in Volume 6 on specific nursing interventions, and chapters in Volume 7 on physiological aspects of nursing.

In the area of nursing care delivery, Violet H. Barkauskas analyzes research on home health care, and Phyllis R. Schultz and Karen L. Miller examine nursing administration research from a general perspective. In the section on nursing education, as in previous volumes, there is a focus on areas of specialized clinical education. Marguerite R. Kinney reviews research on critical care nursing education, and JoAnn S. Jamann-Riley examines research education.

Research on the profession of nursing includes a chapter by Joan G. Turner on Acquired Immune Deficiency Syndrome (AIDS).

In the area of other research, one chapter is included. Bonnie J. Garvin and Carol W. Kennedy review research on nurse–patient communication. In this section we are interested particularly in including international nursing research; we have targeted chapters in future volumes that will be focused on nursing research in other countries. We welcome your suggestions for authors from other countries to review the nursing research in that country.

The success of the *Annual Review* over the past several years has been enhanced by the contributions of the distinguished Advisory Board. We always welcome their suggestions and appreciate their advice and support. We also acknowledge the critiques of anonymous reviewers and the editorial and clerical assistance provided by support staff at Case Western Reserve University, the University of Kansas, and the University of Washington.

As always, we welcome readers' comments and suggestions for shaping the upcoming volumes, including identifying potential chapter contributors. Please let us know your interests in contributing to the series and your comments on this volume.

Contributors

Violet H. Barkauskas, Ph.D.
School of Nursing
The University of Michigan
Ann Arbor, Michigan

Elizabeth M. Burns, Ph.D.
College of Nursing
The Ohio State University
Columbus, Ohio

Carolyn E. Carlson, Ph.D.
Department of Nursing
Cedarville College
Cedarville, OH, and
Rehabilitation Institute
  of Chicago
Chicago, Illinois

Marie J. Cowan, Ph.D.
School of Nursing
University of Washington
Seattle, Washington

Bonnie J. Garvin, Ph.D.
College of Nursing
The Ohio State University
Columbus, Ohio

JoAnn S. Jamann-Riley, Ed.D.
School of Nursing
Columbia University
New York, New York

Carol W. Kennedy, Ph.D.
College of Nursing
The Ohio State University
Columbus, Ohio

Rosemarie B. King, Ph.D.
Rehabilitation Institute
  of Chicago
Chicago, Illinois

Marguerite Kinney, D.N.Sc.
School of Nursing
University of Alabama at
  Birmingham
Birmingham, Alabama

Karen L. Miller, Ph.D.
The Children's Hospital and
  School of Nursing
  University of Colorado
  Health Sciences Center
Denver, Colorado

Kathleen A. O'Connell, Ph.D.
Midwest Research Institute and
School of Nursing
University of Kansas Medical
  Center
Kansas City, Kansas

Phyllis R. Schultz, Ph.D.
School of Nursing
University of Washington
Seattle, Washington

Joan G. Turner, D.S.N.
School of Nursing
University of Alabama at
  Birmingham
Birmingham, Alabama

Forthcoming

ANNUAL REVIEW OF
NURSING RESEARCH, Volume 9

Tentative Contents

PART I

Research on Nursing Practice

Chapter 1

Cardiovascular Nursing Research

MARIE J. COWAN
SCHOOL OF NURSING
UNIVERSITY OF WASHINGTON

CONTENTS

To begin this review, a historical overview of the development of cardiovascular nursing research is presented. These comments are followed by discussion of the conceptual classification system used in the current evaluation of the research literature.

Three investigators have written reviews of cardiovascular nursing research (Foster, Kloner, & Stengrevics, 1984; Kinney, 1984, 1985) or critical care nursing (Lindsey, 1982, 1983, 1984). These reviewers concluded that cardiovascular nurse researchers have been described as failing to pursue a distinct line of investigation as seen in the number of

3

isolated studies on various topics. Also, most studies were on technical aspects of nursing care without conceptualization and development of a theoretical model. Thus, in the early 1970s, most cardiovascular nursing research had been aimed at electrocardiographic studies that were for the most part descriptive. Many studies were done on (a) endotracheal suctioning, (b) hemodynamic monitoring, and (c) recording of cardiovascular variables such as heart rate, blood pressure, pulmonary artery pressure, pulmonary artery end-diastolic pressure, and cardiac output, with the patient in different positions. The sample sizes were small, and few of the investigators continued to follow a single line of inquiry. Most of the reports were single, isolated investigations.

Beginning in the 1980s, the development of knowledge in cardiovascular nursing mirrored the development of nursing science throughout the country. In an attempt to specify the nature of cardiovascular nursing science, the studies in this review were evaluated according to their fit with the fields of study in the conceptualization of nursing science at the University of Washington School of Nursing (de Tornyay, 1977). In this conceptualization two of the fields are concerned with phenomena or human responses related to individuals' and families' adaptations to wellness and illness. The third field is the study of supporting and nonsupporting environments. The fourth, clinical therapeutics, deals with the therapeutic or change process, which is nursing care.

The purpose of this review was to classify cardiovascular nursing studies into the four fields of nursing science defined above. The aim was to identify and describe aggregations of studies in which phenomena were examined according to an organized conceptualization of cardiovascular nursing science. In the past, with a few notable exceptions (e.g., Sivarajan et al., 1981), there were no aggregations of studies in which nurse investigators have examined similar physiological, psychological, or social phenomena related to care of the cardiovascular patient. The majority of studies to date have been diverse; consequently, the contributions to nursing knowledge remain fragmentary.

METHODS OF REVIEW

The search for cardiovascular nursing research was done in several ways. A bibliographic citation list for the years 1977 through 1987 was generated by MEDLARS II, producing a total of 764 citations. The journals or proceedings listed for the MEDLARS search were *Communicating Nursing Research*; *Heart & Lung*; *Cardiovascular Nursing*; *Nursing Research*; *Research in Nursing & Health*; *Western Journal of Nursing Research*; *The Journal of Cardiovascular Nursing*; and *Progress in Cardiovascular Nursing*. The MEDLARS bibliographic citation list was perused to identify publications likely to be research reports and articles deemed appropriate for the review. Copies of published papers and abstracts were also obtained through correspondence with known nurse investigators in the field of cardiovascular nursing. Eighteen cardiovascular nurse scientists were sent letters asking for reprints of their research or their curriculum vitae. Eleven responded to the query and sent a total of 151 articles.

Four criteria were developed for use in evaluating the published papers: (a) the inclusion of a theoretical framework; (b) a clear description of the methodology including design, sample, instrument, and analytical procedures; (c) methods of analysis appropriate to the data; and (d) conclusions based on the results of the study. Of the 764 bibliographic citations from the MEDLARS search, 126 articles fit these criteria. Thus, 277 articles were read for this review: 126 articles from the MEDLARS search and 151 articles from the query of cardiovascular nurse scientists. Of the 277 articles that were read, 138 articles were used as references in this review.

The 138 articles were examined on the following dimensions: purpose statements; phenomena measured; populations (persons with myocardial infarctions, coronary bypass graft surgery, hypertension, valvular surgery); sample size; interventions; results; and classification into fields of study. After all of the articles were evaluated, the collective responses were summarized.

INDIVIDUAL ADAPTATION TO CORONARY ARTERY DISEASE

This field of nursing science is the study of responses of individuals in states of wellness and illness. The focus is on the description of responses of individuals to cardiovascular disease and the means used by individuals for promoting health, preventing disease and disability, fostering recovery from illness, and achieving rehabilitation to optimal functioning.

Health Promotion and Prevention of Disease

Studies aimed at modification of risk factors of coronary artery disease are in the evolving stage of cardiovascular nursing research. These investigators commonly tested multivariate models that incorporated concepts from social psychology theory as mediating variables and behaviors such as lowering blood pressure, reducing stress, increasing exercise, decreasing smoking, and lowering the cholesterol and/or calories in the diet as the outcome variables.

Murdaugh and Hinshaw (1986) tested a model based on theories of social learning and health belief to modify behavior regarding cardiovascular risk factors. The model explained 46% of the variance for exercise and only 7% for smoking behavior. Pender and Pender (1986) used Fishbein's (1980) theory of reasoned action as the conceptual framework. Attitudes, subjective norms, and weight affected intentions to engage in regular exercise. Attitudes, weight, and perceived health status were the principal determinants of intention to eat a diet consistent with weight control. Only attitude was associated with intention to manage stress. Concept development and methodology in both of these studies were excellent. One limitation is that the samples were predominantly white, college-educated, healthy adults. In the Murdaugh and Hinshaw study, only 25% smoked and 65% already were engaged in an exercise program. Thus these a priori activities in the sample probably influenced the small effect size noted in the results.

Other studies of risk factors have been descriptive in design. Gentry, Baider, Oude-Weme, Musch, and Gary (1983) described the Type A and Type B personality differences in patients coping with acute myocardial infarction. Becker et al. (1986) studied smoking behavior among hospital nurses. More recently, Becker and Levine (1987) examined family history of disease and the influence of myocardial infarction of a sibling on the behaviors of unaffected siblings. Brothers and sisters in the aggregate did not perceive their own high relative risk for coronary artery disease. Neither did they change their smoking habits, body weight, dietary salt or fat intake, self-reported stress levels, or exercise patterns significantly in the 4 months following the coronary artery disease event in the sibling. Studies by Becker and associates are good examples of methods appropriate to analyses of risk factors of coronary artery disease.

In summary, identification of the personality factors that influence behavior modification is an area of research of importance to society. Coronary artery disease remains the major cause of morbidity and mortality in the United States. Modification of risk factors for atherosclerosis in the young, the healthy, and those persons with ischemic heart disease could lower the morbidity and mortality rates over time. The risk factors have been identified, but the social–psychological mediating variables inherent in long-term behavior change have yet to be described.

Recovery from Illness and Rehabilitation

These studies can be categorized into adaptation after myocardial infarction, coronary bypass surgery, and hypertension.

Myocardial infarction. Representative examples of studies in this group include assessment of the acute event and assessment of the person's activities of daily living after the event. Cardiac response to myocardial infarction has been described in studies of electrocardiographic responses of persons after myocardial infarction. Jouve, Puddu, and Torresani (1982) and Johnson and Cowan (1986) investigated the electrical systolic duration (QTc) of patients 3 days after acute myocardial infarction. Johnson and Cowan (1986) reported that persons who had out-of-the-hospital ventricular fibrillation with or without acute myocardial infarction had significantly longer QTc intervals than persons with acute myocardial infarction. However, the QTc interval as a criterion to predict sudden cardiac arrest was not a very sensitive measure.

Cowan, Reichenbach, Bruce, and Fisher (1982) estimated the size of the myocardial infarction by electrocardiography. The size of the myocardial infarction, estimated by the initial abnormal depolarization of the QRS waveform (IAD), was correlated highly to the size of the myocardial infarction measured by pathological analysis postmortem. This study was replicated in another independent sample of 55 patients (Cowan, Bruce, & Reichenbach, 1986), and the electrocardiographic variable was used in a randomized clinical trial as a noninvasive clinical measure of infarct size (Cowan, Hindman, Ritchie, & Cerqueira, 1987). Estimations of infarct size are used to evaluate therapy and to predict prognostic outcomes such as cardiogenic shock (Cowan, 1981). In another study Cowan, Bruce, and Reichenbach (1984) showed that the size of inferior myocardial infarctions can be estimated by changes seen in late depolarization, that is, after the peak of the R wave. Lastly, the variable, IAD, can be used reliably for diagnosis of acute myocardial infarction as well as estimation of infarct size (Cowan, Bruce, Van Winkle, Davidson, & Killpack, 1985). Although a valid, reliable, noninvasive estimate of infarct size is highly significant, the main problem is the expense of the technological and software transfer of Cowan's programs for use in practice.

One of the most studied activities of daily living by nurses is the return to sexual activity after an acute myocardial infarction. Classic studies have been done by nurses on heart rate and blood pressure responses to sexual activity after an acute myocardial infarction (Johnston, Cantwell, Watt, & Fletcher, 1978; Larson, McNaughton, Kennedy, & Mansfield, 1980). Heart rate responses to sexual activity and stair climbing were similar for a group of men with coronary artery disease and a group of men with no heart disease. The maximal systolic blood pressure was similar between the two groups during sexual activity (Larson et al., 1980). This study supported the clinical use of a two-flight stair-climbing test, 10 minutes of rapid walking followed by a climb of two flights of stairs in 10 seconds, as a physiologic test of readiness to resume sexual activity after an acute myocardial infarction. Johnston et al. (1978) showed that the absolute frequency of sexual intercourse before and after the cardiac event was decreased significantly in the myocardial infarction group; however, there was no difference in frequency reported by the patients who had coronary bypass graft surgery.

One result of this research on adaptation to acute myocardial infarction is that the size of the myocardial infarction can be measured reliably, validly, and noninvasively by an electrocardiogram, and patients safely can assume low-level exercise after an acute myocardial infarction. The size of the infarct can be used to evaluate therapy and predict prognosis. Prescriptions for low-level activity can be made after a myocardial infarction, specifically for resumption of sexual activity, based on evaluation of a two-flight stair-climbing test or a low-level treadmill test. If the patient can complete the test without dyspnea or angina, presumably other activities that require the same or less metabolic work as sexual activity can be resumed.

Coronary Artery Bypass Graft Surgery.   Studies in this group have been focused on physical as well as psychosocial responses to having coronary artery bypass surgery. The topics have included expectations of the surgery, decision making by the patient and family for the surgery, the desired details of the preoperative teaching, the incidence of postcardiotomy delirium, the physical and psychosocial functioning related to the early phases of rehabilitation, and quality of life after surgery.

Gortner, Gilliss, Moran, Sparacino, and Kenneth (1985) identified the expectations of treatment that influenced patient and family decisions in the choice of treatment for coronary artery disease. The investigators used two groups: patients who underwent coronary bypass surgery and patients who were treated for coronary artery disease without surgery. In the two groups, 57 of 69 expectations were realized. Dimensions of expectations were: prolonging life and preventing myocardial infarction, freedom from pain, improved quality of life, increased exercise, return to work, travel, and return to former activities.

Gilliss, Sparacino, Gortner, and Kenneth (1985) described the major elements of decision making for medical or surgical treatment for coronary artery disease as: (a) severity of illness; (b) events leading to the decision for treatment; and (c) features of the decision for treatment. Coronary bypass graft surgery was the final option for surgical patients after they had tried medical management. Dietary adjustments or exercise were alternative treatments in a small percentage (6–8%) of the patients. Patients chose their own preference for treatment. Most of the patients (67% of the medical and 56% of the surgical patients) indicated they made an independent decision in selecting a treatment option. Cardiologists were the decision makers for 15% of the surgical patients.

Gortner, Rankin, and Wolfe (1988) described the recovery of persons older than 70 years. Exacerbation of previous illness, such as emphysema, diverticulosis, atrial fibrillation, and associated medication toxicity, were at a high incidence upon going home after coronary bypass graft surgery. Coping strategies after surgery revealed a tendency to avoid rather than to express conflicts. Older adults also had significantly lower anger–hostility scores than did younger patients. Perceived self-efficacy for cardiac rehabilitation increased during the first postoperative month at home, with large gains made by patients in the area of perceived confidence in walking ability, general exertion, climbing, and lifting.

Miller and Shada (1978) interviewed 19 adult open-heart surgery patients as to the information included or not included in preoperative instruction they identified as important to recovery. The investigators found that subjects had the greatest difficulty with the respiratory aspect of their care postoperatively. Subjects indicated specific needs for more information about the endotracheal tube, the ventilator, mucus suctioning, deep breathing and coughing, and chest tube removal. Patients experienced transient, primarily depressive, nonpsychotic postoperative mood changes unrelated to preoperative information.

By 1982, Miller, Wikoff, McMahon, Garrett, and Johnson (1982) had developed a tool to measure health attitudes of patients with cardiac disease toward performing prescribed behaviors of their medical regimen. Two groups of subjects with heart disease were used to evaluate validity and reliability of the Miller Attitude Scale. One sample included 480 members of Mended Hearts, Inc., and a second consisted of 35 patients diagnosed with a first myocardial infarction. The Miller Attitude Scale was one of the first measurements with tested psychometrics developed for the cardiac population.

Sadler (1981) studied the relationship of incidence, degree, and duration of postcardiotomy delirium to age of the patient, time on cardiopulmonary bypass, mean arterial pressure on bypass, intensive care unit time, and body temperature postoperatively. The sample consisted of 50 open-heart surgical patients. Manifestations of delirium were experienced by 72% of the sample. The incidence of postcardiotomy delirium was related to blood pressure on bypass, age, and temperature on the third postoperative day. Using these variables as well as temperature on the first postoperative day, delirium accurately was predicted in 76% of the patients. Degree of postcardiotomy delirium was related to age and time in the intensive care unit. Duration of delirium was related to age, ICU time, and temperature on the third postoperative day.

O'Connor (1983) reported on physical and psychosocial functioning related to the early phases of rehabilitation following coronary artery bypass surgery. Although a patient's perceptions of his health improved after surgery, there was little improvement in physical and psychosocial functioning, and vocational functioning declined. Energy expenditure on postoperative leisure activities was related to fear of injury. Preoperative psychosocial functioning, depression, and postoperative perception of health explained postoperative psychosocial functioning.

Penckoser and Holm (1984) studied the relationship of coronary bypass graft surgery and quality of life. The patients viewed their future life satisfaction to be better than their life satisfaction prior to open-heart surgery. Further, they reported a decrease in the level of angina, an increase in the level of physical activity, and increased satisfaction with family life, social life, and sexual life following surgery. This study is a classic because it is one of the earliest nursing studies on quality of life after coronary bypass graft surgery. Most of the studies on quality of life after myocardial infarction or coronary bypass graft surgery have been done by scientists who were not nurses (Cowan, in press).

In summary, studies have been focused on individuals and have included physical as well as psychological responses to having coronary artery bypass surgery. The nurse investigators of the early 1980s who studied adaptation to coronary artery bypass surgery, for the most part, published single articles. Representative examples were the studies of O'Connor (1983), Sadler (1981), Penckoser and Holm (1984), Miller and Shada (1978), and Miller et al. (1982). Gortner is one of the few nurse researchers who has established a program of research centered on the adaptation of the individual and family after coronary artery bypass surgery (Gilliss et al., 1985; Gortner et al., 1985; Gortner et al., 1988). The methodologies of all of the above studies were well designed and appropriate to the research questions.

Hypertension. The underlying psychological and social mechanisms that affect human responses to hypertension now are being clarified through projects of several investigators. Nakagawa-Kogan, Garber, Jarrett, Egan, and Hendershot (1988) studied the effects of biofeedback/self-management on borderline hypertension (diastolic blood pressure of 90–105 mm Hg). Through discriminant analyses, they were able to determine that those people with hypertension who were not able to learn biofeedback to lower their blood pressure had higher self-reported scores of psychologic distress on anger and anxiety. These persons also had higher systolic blood pressure than the other hypertensive persons. Earlier Egan, Nakagawa-Kogan, Garber, and Jarrett (1983) had reported that a relationship existed between psychological distress, life changes, and subsequent control of hypertension.

Other noteworthy projects were the prospective study of 88 diagnosed hypertensive patients (Given, Given, & Simoni, 1978) and the relationship of Type A behavior patterns to hypertension among inner-city blacks (Smyth, Hansell, Sparacino, & Strodbeck, 1978). Sparacino, Hansell, and Smyth (1979) and Sparacino, Ronchi, Brenner, Kuhn, and Flesch (1982) described the relationship of blood pressure to hostility, anxiety, and Type A coronary-prone behavior. In summary, the amount of nursing research on hypertension has been inadequate. More studies are needed on risk-factor modification and different interventions such as low-sodium diet, relaxation techniques, loss of weight, and other techniques used to lower blood pressure.

FAMILY ADAPTATION TO CORONARY ARTERY DISEASE

The social unit of the family is influential to risk factor reduction and support after cardiovascular disease. What is known about families' adaptations to the immediate impact of cardiac disease results from studies of adult families after myocardial infarction or cardiac surgery. Gilliss et al. (1985) compared the events leading to treatment for two sets of subjects: coronary artery bypass graft patients and families, and medically controlled coronary artery disease patients and families. The investigators reported that considerably more disruption of family patterns was seen in the bypass group and concluded that the bypass families, in contrast to their medically controlled counterparts, viewed the surgery as a crisis. The stressor most frequently identified by the families was waiting for surgery. Another major stressor reported by spouses was a lack of control of hospital events. Spouses lacked the privacy they believed they needed, mainly to be able to cry.

During the recovery period, spouses often were frightened of the responsibility of caring for the patient and identified the early days when the patient was home from the hospital as being the most difficult and frightening. Patient and spouse would argue over what the patient could and should do. The conflict was described generally to grow from the early acts of the spouse in protecting the patient (Gilliss, 1984; Gilliss & Hauck, in press).

Gortner and Zyzanski (1988) reported a bioethical study to measure values and the choice of treatment, in particular the choice of surgical treatment for heart disease. The specific aims were to determine which moral values predominated in the sample of bypass and valve replacement patients and families, to confirm the relation of individual or patient values to those of family values as represented by the spouse, and to establish the validity of an inventory. The statements were based on the moral principles of autonomy, beneficence, and nonmaleficence. The results indicated that families valued autonomy significantly more than beneficence or nonmaleficence, irrespective of the type of surgical procedure, setting, study status, or gender.

Other notable studies on family adapation to coronary artery disease were Balda and Cohen (1980); Becker and Levine (1987); Bramwell (1986); Bramwell and Whall (1986); Doerr and Jones (1979); Dracup, Guzy, Taylor, and Barry (1986); Gortner et al. (1988); Gortner, Baldwin, and Shortridge (1980); Hilbert (1985); and Nyamathi (1987). Representative examples discussed are Bramwell and Whall (1986), Dracup et al. (1986), and Gortner et al. (1988).

Bramwell and Whall (1986) studied the effects of role clarity and empathy on support role, performance, and anxiety. The purpose of the study was to examine wives' anxiety in response to the husband's first myocardial infarction. From the wives' perceptions and interpretations of their support roles, the women described the relationship of their ability to act supportively to the degree of their husbands' anxiety. The results supported two hypotheses: support role performance has a direct negative effect on anxiety, and trait anxiety has a direct positive effect on state anxiety.

Reducing risk also can be accomplished through environmental manipulation. Victims of sudden cardiac illness sometimes survive when cardiopulmonary resuscitation is begun by bystanders. Dracup et al. (1986) used a control trial to evaluate the effect of teaching cardiopulmonary resuscitation (CPR) to the families of high-risk cardiac patients. Although no differences were seen in family members' depression or anxiety, patients in the treatment groups appeared more anxious than controls at 3 and 6 months after the family intervention. Patient anxiety in the treatment group may have been related to changes in the behaviors of family members. Conceivably, these family members were in a state of alertness to the possibility of cardiac arrest requiring them to initiate CPR, and patients responded to these behavioral changes with increased anxiety levels.

Gortner et al. (1988) tested a nursing intervention based on self-efficacy and family stress theory to help families cope after cardiac surgery. The intervention consisted of educational materials on risk factors and surgical rehabilitation, individual counseling for patient and spouse, and telephone contacts with families for 8 weeks after discharge. The effectiveness of the interventions was assessed through a randomized trial in which 67 prospective bypass and valve surgery patients and their spouses were assigned either to the experimental intervention or conventional care and followed for 6 months. At 3 months postsurgery, the only statistically significant difference between the experimental and control groups was on perceived self-efficacy for tolerating emotional distress. At 6 months, no significant differences were found on individual or family measures. However, the experimental nursing intervention was effective in promoting the spouses' "recovery from the surgery."

From this research, the investigators concluded that families are at high risk for disruption following a cardiac event, especially cardiac surgery. Families need information about the usual nature of the cardiac event and may need special nursing services to maintain their integrity during an episode of cardiac illness. Spouses need preparation for the roles they are expected to perform after discharge. Role preparation should include information about the disease, the impact of the surgery, diet, medication, and smoking, and specific information about activity, including sexual activity.

ENVIRONMENTS: SUPPORTING AND NONSUPPORTING

The research studies related to environments supportive of the cardiovascular patient are very sparse. They deal mainly with three broad categories: transfer of the patient from the critical care unit (Minckley, Burrows, Ehrat, Harper, & Jenkins, 1979; Schwartz & Brenner, 1979; Toth, 1980); the correlation between sleep deprivation and the intensive care unit syndrome (Helton, Gordon, & Nunnery, 1980); and the stress effects on patients in critical care units from procedures performed on others (Vanson, Katz, & Krekler, 1980).

Topf (1984) developed a theoretical framework for organizing research according to the health effects from aversive physical aspects of the environment. The framework was substantiated by using the impact of hospital noise upon recovery as an example. Although it was not a research study, supportive theoretical and research literature was cited for substantiating the relationships hypothesized in the framework. Given that research in the field of environments is underdeveloped, Topf's theoretical conceptualization might be a basis for studies on aversive physical aspects of caregiving environments.

CLINICAL THERAPEUTICS

Nursing practice must be influenced and directed by research findings, rather than by beliefs and common behaviors "to get the job done." The focus of most of these studies is a nursing intervention. The evidence from the studies shows knowledge development extending from very technical aspects of nursing care to multidimensional conceptual models on health promotion interventions to be tested. For purposes of discussion, clinical therapeutics is divided into hemodynamic monitoring, endotracheal suctioning, activity prescription, patient education, health promotion interventions, and self-management interventions.

Hemodynamic Monitoring

Research on hemodynamic monitoring has been the most common type of study in cardiovascular nursing. These studies can be divided into the following classifications: (a) the effect of patient position and ventilation on measurements of pulmonary activity and pulmonary artery wedge pressures; (b) the effect of injectable volume and temperature on measurement of thermodilution cardiac output; (c) the effect of automatic versus hand injection of injectate on thermodilution cardiac output; and (d) the effects of position on measurement of thermodilution cardiac output. For brevity, a listing of the many investigators is given followed by a summary of the results from these studies in aggregate.

These investigators looked at the effect of backrest position on the measurement of pulmonary artery and pulmonary artery wedge pressures: Chulay and Miller (1984); Clochesy, Hinshaw, and Oho (1984); Gershan (1983); Grose and Woods (1981); Laulive (1982); Nemens and Woods (1982); O'Quinn and Marini (1983); Kirchhoff, Rebensen-Piano, and Patel (1984); Riedinger and Shellock (1984a); Riedinger, Shellock, and Swan (1981); Shinn, Woods, and Huseby (1979); Woods, Grose, and Laurent-Bopp (1982); and Woods and Mansfield (1976). The following investigators looked at the effect of the lateral position on pulmonary artery and pulmonary artery wedge pressures: Kennedy and Crawford (1984); Whitman (1982); Keating, Bolyard, Eichler, and Reed (1986); Daily and Mersch (1987); and Wild (1984).

A large number of investigators studied the effect of injectate volume and temperature on measurement of thermodilution of cardiac output: Armengol, Man, and Balsys (1981); Bilfinger, Chung-Yuan, and Anagnostopoulous (1982); Callaghan, Weintraub, and Coran (1976); Grose, Woods, and Laurent (1981); Elkayam, Berkley, and Azen (1983); Hoel (1978); Jansen, Schreuder, and Bogaard (1981); Kadota (1986); Kohanna and Cunningham (1977); Levett and Replogle (1979); Mannesmann and Muller (1980); Merrick, Hessel, and Dillard (1980); Moodie, Feldt, and Kaye (1979); Nelson and Houtchens (1982); Pelletier (1979); Powner and Snyder (1978); Riedinger and Shellock (1984b); Runciman, Isley, and Roberts (1981); Shellock and Riedinger (1983); Shellock, Riedinger, and Bateman (1983); Snyder and Powner (1982); Stawicki, Holford, and Michelson (1979); Stetz, Miller, and Kelly (1982); Swan and Ganz (1983); Tajiri, Katsuya, and Okamoto (1984); Vennix, Nelson, and Pierpont (1984); Weil (1977); and Woog and McWilliam (1983). Dizon, Gezan, and Barash (1977) and Manifold (1984) studied the effect of automatic versus hand injection of ejectate on thermodilution cardiac output. Grose and Woods (1981), Kleven (1984), and Whitman, Howaniak, and Verga (1982) studied the effects of position on thermodilution cardiac output.

The summaries of findings based on these studies on hemodynamic measurements would indicate several nursing practice implications. Compared to the flat position, reproducible pulmonary artery and pulmonary artery wedge pressures can be obtained in most cases at backrest elevation of 60 degrees or 30 degrees. There are some individuals who do have changes in pressure with backrest elevation; thus it is important to determine whether there is a difference for each patient before assuming that there is no difference for multiple measurements. Compared to the flat position, reproducible pulmonary artery and pulmonary artery wedge pressures can be obtained in most patients in the 90-degree lateral position using the midsternum as the zero reference point.

For those patients with mechanical ventilation without pulmonary end-expiration pressure (PEEP), pulmonary artery and pulmonary artery wedge pressures should be measured at end-expiration on and off the ventilator to determine differences. If no differences are found, then pressures can be measured at end-expiration on the ventilator.

Five to ten ml of room temperature injectate provide accurate measurements of thermodilution cardiac output in most patients.

These volumes apply to room temperatures that are between 19 degrees and 25 degrees C and to catheters that are interfaced with computers with computation constants for room temperature. Automatic injection of injectate produces less variation in thermodilution cardiac output than hand injection.

Compared to the flat position, reproducible thermodilution cardiac output measurements can be obtained in most patients at backrest elevations of 20 degrees or less and in lateral positions. Cardiac output varies with the phases of the respiratory cycle; thus injection should be made at consistent times during the cycle.

Endotracheal Suctioning

A second example of research on nursing therapeutics pertains to studies of endotracheal suctioning. Both human and dog models have been used. An example of an investigator who has built a program of research around endotracheal sunctioning is Powaser (Adlkofer & Powaser, 1978; Skelley, Deeren, & Powaser, 1980; Woodburne & Powaser, 1980). In addition, other investigators such as Buchanan and Baun (1986) and Goodnough (1985) have contributed to knowledge on the effects of this procedure. Most of these investigators have focused their techniques on prevention of a fall in arterial oxygen tension (PaO$_2$) as a consequence of suctioning. A thorough review of the research dealing with endotracheal suctioning can be found in a review article by Rudy, Baun, Stone, and Turner (1986).

Activity Prescription

The accepted course of care for the patient recovering from an acute myocardial infarction or coronary bypass graft surgery in the 1980s is characterized by an early resumption of physical activity, a decrease in imposed invalidism, and early discharge from the hospital. Early ambulation has been demonstrated to be desirable, feasible, cost-effective, and safe. Several nurse investigators have contributed to knowledge in support of early ambulation after acute myocardial infarction (Ahrens, Kinney, & Carter, 1983; Beeby & Cowan, 1984; Hathaway & Geden, 1983; Holm, Fink, Chrisman, Reitz, & Ashley, 1985; Johnston, 1984; Lerman, Bruce, Sivarajan, Pettet, & Trimble, 1976; Lindskog & Sivarajan, 1982; Mansfield, Sivarajan, & Bruce,

1978; Ott et al., 1983; Sivarajan et al., 1981; Sivarajan & Bruce, 1981; Sivarajan, Lerman, Mansfield, & Bruce, 1977).

Sivarajan et al. (1981) accomplished one of the key research projects to show that an in-hospital exercise program of early ambulation and treadmill testing at a low level, an approximate 3 metabolic equivalent (MET) level, did not demonstrate any significant harmful effects after an acute myocardial infarction. One MET is the patient's approximate oxygen consumption while sitting quietly in a chair. This research was done using careful, systematic methods such that the reader can have confidence in the results. The study was at the "cutting edge" for its time because low-level exercise treadmill tests were not given then to a patient with an acute myocardial infarction because of a fear of the test being too stressful. Low-level exercise testing is now common practice. Sivarajan is an example of a nurse researcher who has a continuous program of research and has contributed to the development of knowledge on activity and exercise prescription after an acute myocardial infarction (Lerman et al., 1976; Lindskog & Sivarajan, 1982; Mansfield et al., 1978; Ott et al., 1983; Sivarajan et al., 1977, 1981; Sivarajan & Bruce, 1981). Johnston's findings (1984) supported the findings of Sivarajan and associates that low-level exercise after an acute myocardial infarction is a safe measure and may be predictive of prognosis upon discharge.

Holm et al. (1985) studied health beliefs, health motivation, perceptions of illness, perceptions of resusceptibility, efficacy of treatment, barriers to treatment, cues to taking health-related action, patient satisfaction, social support, and self-motivation in a group of cardiac patients who initiated and completed an outpatient cardiac exercise program. Scores on the measures revealed subjects to be externally controlled, satisfied with the program and staff, recipients of social support, and self-motivated. The most significant relationships were between perceptions of severity of illness and general health motivation, perceptions of severity and resusceptibility, cues to taking health-related action and satisfaction with program staff, and satisfaction with the program and the program staff.

Ahrens et al. (1983) and Hathaway and Geden (1983) have studied the effects of leg exercise programs. Hathaway and Geden (1983) compared the effects of active, passive, and isometric exercise programs and a rest program control on energy expenditure (oxygen consumption), heart rate, respiratory rate, and blood pressure. In general, the results indicated that on oxygen consumption and heart rate the isometric and active programs were comparable and significantly more demanding than either the passive or rest programs.

Cardiovascular nurse researchers also have studied the physiological effects of activities such as bathing after an acute myocardial infarction. Johnston, Watt, and Fletcher (1981) studied physiological responses before, during, and after three types of baths in 10 patients with uncomplicated acute myocardial infarction during the immediate 3-to-5-day period of hospitalization. Shower activity demanded greater energy, that is, oxygen consumption, than either tub or bed bathing. The peak pressure rate product (peak systolic blood pressure × heart rate divided by 100) was greater for showering when compared to bed bathing but not to tub bathing. None of the patients complained of angina, and there were no arrhythmias during any of the baths.

Winslow, Lane, and Gaffney (1985) also measured physiological responses before, during, and after three types of baths in 18 patients who were 5 to 17 days postacute myocardial infarction and in 22 control patients. For the patients oxygen consumption during shower activity was similar to the other types of bathing; the patients had significantly lower oxygen consumption during bathing than did the control subjects. The patients' peak heart rates were higher than anticipated with the level of exertion and sometimes exceeded the target heart rate used in previous discharge exercise testing. Winslow and associates' findings showed that the physiological cost of three types of baths were similar, and thus many cardiac patients could take a tub bath or shower earlier in their hospitalization than has been the usual practice. However, energy expenditure associated with type of bathing after an acute myocardial infarction is an area in which more research is needed, given that Winslow and associates' results do not agree with those of Johnston et al. (1981).

Patient Education

The studies designed to test the effects of teaching have been focused on the differences between structured and unstructured teaching with the use of compliance or adherence as a dependent variable. These studies have taken place both in the acute-care setting and upon discharge under the auspices of cardiac rehabilitation.

Steele and Ruzicki (1987) demonstrated that inpatient cardiac teaching programs can be effective for short-term outcomes. Patients learned information that prepared them to deal with postoperative experiences such as ambulation, exercise, resumption of sexual activities, and symptoms indicating lack of tolerance for activities. The areas that showed limited knowledge gain were those that required long-term behavioral change, such as stress modification and dietary changes. These findings are important when considered in light of decreases in length of stay in hospitals and increases in acuity levels of hospitalized patients. Inpatient teaching should be limited to what is possible and reasonable for the staff to accomplish and for patients to learn.

Toth (1980) compared the effects of structured versus unstructured teaching on patient anxiety on transfer from the coronary care unit. Twenty myocardial infarction patients were studied; half received structured pretransfer teaching designed to orient them to differences in the environment and care in the progressive unit. All patients received the unstructured pretransfer teaching by the coronary care unit nurses. The anxiety level of subjects who received the structured pretransfer teaching was significantly lower than the anxiety level of control subjects on the physiological parameters measured: systolic blood pressure the day and time of transfer, and heart rates the day and time of transfer.

Cardiac rehabilitation programs are intended to assist patients who have experienced myocardial infarction to return to normal lives and to establish changes in lifestyle by modifying risk factors of coronary artery disease, such as smoking, hypertension, hyperlipidemia, stress, and obesity. The behavioral changes include cessation of smoking, low-sodium diets, low-calorie diets, habitual regular exercise, stress reduction techniques, and low-cholesterol diets.

Sivarajan et al. (1983) studied the effects of three interventions on risk factor modification. The interventions were a teaching and counseling program, conventional medical and nursing management, and a teaching and counseling program with exercise prescription. The classes were planned around specific topics: (a) the development of atherosclerosis, myocardial infarction, angina, and other symptoms; (b) coronary artery disease risk factors; (c) nutrition; (d) dietary changes; (e) exercise and activity; (f) stress and relaxation; (g) return to work and sexual activity; and (h) emotional reactions to myocardial infarction. The dependent variables were cigarette smoking, dietary intake of selected food items, and weight changes. The sample was 258 patients who were randomized into one of the three groups. The results showed no statistically significant difference among the interventions on any of the dependent variables. In terms of overall behavioral changes, the teaching and counseling program on risk factors demonstrated only limited effectiveness. The approach to teaching and counseling was to provide accurate and practical information to patients who had made the decision to implement changes in their diet or smoking habits. The education was provided primarily in a group approach and did not give attention to individualized risk factor strategies. Sivarajan et al. concluded that this approach has major limitations because acquisition of correct knowledge is only one of the many factors that influence behavior change.

The results of Sivarajan et al. are supported by those of Swain and Steckel (1981) regarding problems of nonadherence to the treatment of hypertension and consequent poor blood pressure control. One hundred and fifteen patients were assigned randomly to one of three treatment modalities: routine clinic care, patient education, and contingency contracting. They were followed over four clinic visits. Patient education was not effective in lowering blood pressure. In fact, assignment to this treatment showed a dropout rate higher than that for patients receiving only routine clinic care. However, contingency contracting was an effective intervention strategy for improving patient knowledge, adhering to requests for medical care, and decreasing diastolic blood pressures.

The evidence from these studies shows that structured teaching is better than nonstructured teaching in terms of knowledge scores. However, structured teaching alone does not affect health behaviors. Gregor (1981) found that a systematic approach to teaching increased posttest scores in patients with ischemic heart disease. Also, Marshall, Penckofer, and Llewellyn (1986) studied a convenience sample of two comparable groups of patients who had coronary artery bypass surgery. The sample size was 64 patients. One group was educated by an unstructured method; the other group received structured teaching with a guide developed by nurses experienced in open-heart surgery. Knowledge was assessed before instituting teaching, upon discharge from the hospital, and 6 weeks after discharge. Both groups had higher total knowledge scores after surgery. In addition, the patients who had structured teaching had higher total compliance scores than those who had unstructured teaching, and walked more blocks after surgery than those who received routine teaching.

Mills, Barnes, Rodell, and Terry (1985) asked many of the same questions as Marshall et al. (1986). A sample of 342 patients with ischemic heart disease was assigned to an inpatient cardiac education program consisting of five daily 1-hour classes. The specific aims of the study were to evaluate the impact of a patient education program on the patient's knowledge regarding his or her illness and to identify obstacles to compliance behavior after discharge. The study was conducted over a 2-year period. Patients were assigned randomly such that one group received a pretest and a posttest assessment of knowledge and the second group received only the posttest assessment. The data included assessment of an individual's knowledge of his or her illness, selected sociodemographic information, measures of general intelligence, problem-solving ability, and motivation to alter risk factors. The results showed that indicators of motivation were most highly correlated with compliance.

In summary, some knowledge about patient education and coronary artery disease has been gained from these few studies. First, patients deal poorly with lectures about cardiac anatomy and physiology and appear to learn better the specific recommendations for what to do to manage their heart disease, and when. The timing of providing information to the patient appears to be critical. Information provided in the hospital needs to be addressed to those care and management problems dealing with the acuity of the disease. Most of the studies focusing on patient education have been limited because of small sample size, lack of randomization, and/or lack of standardization of the intervention, that is, the educational material. However, these limitations were not evident in the studies by Sivarajan et al. (1983), Swain and Steckel (1981), and Mills et al. (1985).

After discharge, education alone does not appear to modify behaviors regarding risk factor reduction or prescription adherence. Despite the excellence of inpatient education programs, behavioral changes are not attained on knowledge alone. Rather the noncognitive domains of learning retention and compliance need to be studied. The studies by Johnson et al. (Johnson, Rice, Fuller, & Endress, 1978) on the value of sensory information and instruction on coping strategies for dealing with major surgeries provide models for future research in cardiovascular nursing. The most effective teaching strategy in the hospital has been a combination of essential specific information about managing the disease effects, effective nursing management, and the individualization of that management for the person under treatment.

Health Promotion Interventions

The studies on patient education paved the way for theoretical models taken from sociology and psychology and modified by nurse scientists for the purposes of behavior modification with respect to risk factors of coronary artery disease. Jordan-Marsh and Neutra (1985) described the relationship of health locus of control scores to changes in physical parameters of 339 participants in a lifestyle change program. The dependent variables included weight, blood pressure, low-density lipoproteins, triglycerides, and the ratio between cholesterol and high-density lipoproteins. Data were collected on admission and upon completion of the 24-day residential program and at a 6-month followup. Differences in health locus of control scores on admission and on discharge were significant. Weight changes at 6 months correlated positively with admission health locus of control composite scores.

McCance, Eutropius, Jacobs, and Williams (1985) studied a preventive nursing intervention to reduce coronary heart disease in a sample of 19 families composed of 58 relatives of young victims of sudden cardiac death. Families were assigned randomly to control and experimental groups. The intervention at 2 to 5 months after death was focused on assessment of health history, health behaviors, health beliefs, informing and educating about coronary artery disease risk factors, and methods for detecting and reducing these factors. The control group received mailed-in questionnaires and no intervention. The subject's reduction of coronary artery risk factors was measured at 7 months by changes in high-risk coronary artery disease behaviors, changes in health beliefs, adherence to screening for serum cholesterol, and blood pressure determination. The intervention was correlated with a significant reduction in alcohol intake. Reductions in high-fat meat consumption were in the desired direction. Greater percentages of subjects in the intervention group obtained blood pressure and cholesterol screening.

Ventura et al. (1984) studied the effectiveness of health promotion interventions. The purpose of the study was to determine whether patients with peripheral vascular disease who participated in an intervention program would improve exercise and foot care habits, reduce smoking, and have fewer related diseases than patients not exposed to the intervention. The intervention was a process/outcome model incorporating concepts from adult learning theory and the use of referent power as a means of promoting health behavior. Eighty-six patients with ankle bracheal pressure indices of less than one on one or both legs were assigned randomly to a study ($n = 44$) group. All patients were assessed on a variety of health-related variables and activities prior to and 26 weeks after enrollment in the study. At the end of 26 weeks there were no significant differences between study and control groups on smoking and foot care, although the results were in the anticipated direction. Study patients who chose to increase their exercise showed greater increase than control patients in frequency, distance, and length of walks. Although behaviors were modified, especially in the area of exercise, the investigators believed that longer interventions on a larger sample were needed. A criticism of the study is that patients who made no change were not included in the analysis for the variable in question. Thus, with a bias toward change, the reported trend in the anticipated direction as caused by the intervention remains questionable.

The construction of multivariate models to test interventions to change behaviors are in the development state in cardiovascular nursing science. The significance of this research direction lies in the fact that coronary artery disease is the major cause of mortality and morbidity in the United States and Europe. Knowledge about effective strategies for the modification or reduction of risk factors for coronary artery disease depends on the development of sophisticated approaches to evaluation research.

Self-Management Interventions

A clinical therapeutic in the development stage is based on the assumption that individuals cognitively can control their own physiological responses and affective states as a form of management of symptoms. Progressive relaxation training, biofeedback, and self-management training have been of interest in cardiac rehabilitation. An example is Bohachick's (1984) study to investigate the effect of progressive relaxation training as a stress management technique for cardiac patients in a cardiac exercise program. The patients received 3 weeks of relaxation training in addition to exercise therapy. A control group of 19 patients was not taught the technique. The posttreatment mean anxiety scores for the treatment group were significantly lower than those of the control group, and the posttest scores for the treatment group were significantly lower for the dimensions of somatization, interpersonal sensitivity, anxiety, and depression than for the control group.

Nakagawa-Kogan et al. (1988) reported that 74% of patients with borderline hypertension cognitively could control their diastolic blood pressures and maintain them under 90 mmHg 50% of the time at home after biofeedback and self-management training. The scores measuring affective states, such as anxiety and depression, were significantly lower after this training. Although biofeedback relaxation techniques to reduce stress have been tested in other populations, they have not been tested extensively in the cardiovascular disease population and merit further research.

FUTURE RESEARCH DIRECTIONS

Given this perspective on the past and present of cardiovascular nursing research, some predictions are offered about knowledge development in the future. Cardiovascular nurse scientists will continue to examine physiological and behavioral human responses in interaction. Conceptual models that integrate the psychological and the physiological responses to cardiovascular disease will be tested in relationship to risk factor modification and interventions to reduce stress and to promote healthy lifestyles. A high priority is research designed to describe the quality of life for patients after myocardial infarction, coronary bypass graft surgery, heart transplant, or sudden cardiac arrest. Fundamental questions about the biophysical and psychosocial indicators of psychosocial phenomena related to adaptation to cardiac disease are in need of investigation. For example, studies on the promotion of health and prevention of cardiac disease in children as well as adults are of significance for society. Further research on nursing therapy in regard to family adaptation to the crises of cardiovascular disease, sudden cardiac death, and heart transplant needs to be done. A challenge for cardiovascular nurse scientists is to do research targeted toward prevention of cardiovascular disease and sudden cardiac death as well as to help patients and families adapt to cardiovascular disease and improve the quality of their lives.

REFERENCES

Adlkofer, R., & Powaser, M. (1978). The effect of endotracheal suctioning on arterial blood gases in patients after cardiac surgery. *Heart & Lung, 7,* 1011–1014.

Ahrens, W., Kinney, M., & Carter, R. (1983). Effects of antistasis footboard exercises on selected measures of exertion. *Heart & Lung, 12,* 366–371.

Armengol, J., Man, G., & Balsys, A. (1981). Effects of the respiratory cycle on cardiac output measurements: Reproducibility of data enhanced by timing the thermodilution injection in dogs. *Critical Care Medicine, 9,* 852–854.

Balda, J., & Cohen, F. (1980). Group sessions: Their effect on distress levels of wives of myocardial infarction patients. *Circulation 62*(III), 172.

Becker, D., & Levine, D. (1987). Risk perception, knowledge, and lifestyles in siblings of people with premature coronary disease. *American Journal of Preventive Medicine, 3,* 45–50.

Becker, D., Myers, A., Facci, M., Weida, S., Swank, R., Levine, D., & Parson, T. (1986). Smoking behavior and attitudes toward smoking among hospital nurses. *American Journal of Public Health, 76,* 1449–1451.

Beeby, B., & Cowan, M. (1984). In-hospital progressive activity: Comparison between myocardial infarction patients with no complications and with out-of-hospital ventricular fibrillation. *Heart & Lung, 13,* 361–365.

Bilfinger, T., Chung-Yuan, L., & Anagnostopoulous, C. (1982). In vitro determination of accuracy of cardiac output measurements by thermal dilution. *Journal of Surgical Research, 33,* 409–414.

Bohachick, P. (1984). Progressive relaxation training in cardiac rehabilitation: Effect on psychologic variables. *Nursing Research, 33,* 283–287.

Bramwell, L. (1986). Wives' experience in the support role after husbands' first myocardial infarction. *Heart & Lung, 15,* 578–584.

Bramwell, L., & Whall, A. (1986). Effect of role clarity and empathy on support role performance and anxiety. *Nursing Research, 35,* 282–287.

Buchanan, L., & Baun, M. (1986). The effect of hyperinflation, inspiratory hold, and oxygenation on cardiopulmonary status during suctioning in a lung injured model. *Heart & Lung, 15,* 127–134.

Callaghan, M., Weintraub, W., & Coran, A. (1976). Assessment of thermodilution cardiac output in small objects. *Journal of Pediatric Surgery, 11,* 629–634.

Chulay, M., & Miller, T. (1984). The effect of backrest elevation on pulmonary artery and pulmonary capillary wedge pressures in patients after cardiac surgery. *Heart & Lung, 13,* 138–140.

Clochesy, J., Hinshaw, A., & Oho, C. (1984). Effect of change of position on pulmonary artery and pulmonary capillary wedge pressures in mechanically ventilated patients. *NITA* (National IV Therapy Association), *7,* 223–225.

Cowan, M. (1981). The relationship between the size of myocardial infarct and the occurrence of cardiogenic shock. *Western Journal of Nursing Research, 3,* 30.

Cowan, M. (in press). A theoretical model of the effects of coronary artery disease on quality of life. *Progress in Cardiovascular Nursing.*

Cowan, M., Bruce, R., & Reichenbach, D. (1984). Estimation of inferobasal myocardial infarct size by late activation abnormalities of the QRS complex. *American Journal of Cardiology, 54*, 726–732.

Cowan, M., Bruce, R., & Reichenbach, D. (1986). Validation of a computerized QRS criterion for estimating myocardial infarction size and correlation with quantitative morphologic measurements. *American Journal of Cardiology, 57*, 60–65.

Cowan, M., Bruce, R., Van Winkle, D., Davidson, L., & Killpack, A. (1985). Comparative accuracy of computerized spatial vectorcardiography and standard electrocardiography for detection of myocardial infarction. *Journal of Electrocardiology, 18*, 111–122.

Cowan, M., Hindman, N., Ritchie, J., & Cerqueira, M. (1987). Estimation of myocardial infarct size by electrocardiographic and radionuclide techniques. *Journal of Electrocardiology, 20*(Suppl.), 78–81.

Cowan, M., Reichenbach, D., Bruce, R., & Fisher, L. (1982). Estimation of myocardial infarct size by digital computer analyses of the VCG. *Journal of Electrocardiology, 15*, 307–316.

Daily, E., & Mersch, J. (1987). Thermodilution cardiac outputs using room and ice temperature injectate: Comparison with the Fick Method. *Heart & Lung, 16*, 294–300.

de Tornyay, R. (1977, April). *A proposal to establish the degree of Doctor of Philosophy in Nursing Science, University of Washington.* Report submitted to the Washington State Post-Secondary Council.

Dizon, C., Gezan, W., & Barash, P. (1977). Hand-held thermodilution cardiac output injector. *Critical Care Medicine, 5*, 210–212.

Doerr, B., & Jones, J. (1979). Effect of family preparation on the state anxiety of the CCU patient. *Nursing Research, 28*, 315–316.

Dracup, K., Guzy, P., Taylor, S., & Barry, J. (1986). Cardiopulmonary resuscitation (CPR) training: Consequences for family members of high risk cardiac patients. *Archives of Internal Medicine, 146*, 1757–1761.

Egan, K., Nakagawa-Kogan, H., Garber, A., & Jarrett, M. (1983). The impact of psychological distress on the control of hypertension. *Journal of Human Stress, 8*, 4–10.

Elkayam, U., Berkley, R., & Azen, S. (1983). Cardiac output by thermodilution technique—Effect of injectate volume and temperature on accuracy reproducibility in the critically ill patient. *Chest, 84*, 418–422.

Fishbein, M. (1980). A theory of reasoned action: Some applications and implications. In H. E. House (Ed.), *Nebraska symposium on motivation* (Vol. 27). Lincoln, NB: University Press.

Foster, S., Kloner, J., & Stengrevics, S. (1984). Cardiovascular nursing research: Past, present and future. *Heart & Lung, 13*, 111–116.

Gentry, W., Baider, L., Oude-Weme, J., Musch, S., & Gary, H. (1983). Type A, B difference in coping with acute myocardial infarction: Further considerations. *Heart & Lung, 12*, 212–214.

Gershan, J. (1983). Effect of positive end-expiratory pressures on pulmonary capillary wedge pressure. *Heart & Lung, 12*, 143–148.

Gilliss, C. (1984). Reducing family stress during and after coronary artery bypass surgery. *Nursing Clinics of North America, 19*, 103–112.

Gilliss, C., & Hauck, W. (in press). Improving family functioning after cardiac surgery: A randomized trial. *Nursing Research.*

Gilliss, C., Sparacino, P., Gortner, S., & Kenneth, H. (1985). Events leading to the treatment of coronary artery disease: Implications for nursing care. *Heart & Lung, 14,* 350–356.

Given, C., Given, B., & Simoni, L. (1978). Association of knowledge and perception of medications with compliance and health states among hypertension patients: A prospective study. *Research in Nursing & Health, 1,* 76–80.

Goodnough, S. (1985). The effects of oxygen and hyperinflation on arterial oxygen tension after intertracheal suctioning. *Heart & Lung, 14,* 11–17.

Gortner, S., Baldwin, A., & Shortridge, L. (1980). Ethical influences of family decisions regarding election of treatment. *Western Journal of Nursing Research, 2,* 508–512.

Gortner, S., Gilliss, C., Moran, J., Sparacino, P., & Kenneth, H. (1985). Expected and realized benefits from coronary bypass surgery in relation to severity of illness. *Cardiovascular Nursing, 21,* 13–18.

Gortner, S., Gilliss, C., Shinn, J., Sparacino, P., Rankin, S., Leavitt, M., Price, M., & Hudes, M. (1988). Improving recovery following cardiac surgery: A randomized clinical trial. *Journal of Advanced Nursing, 13,* 649–661.

Gortner, S., Rankin, S., & Wolfe, M. (1988). Elders' recovery from cardiac surgery. *Progress in Cardiovascular Nursing, 3*(2), 54–61.

Gortner, S., & Zyzanski, S. (1988). Values and the choice of treatment: A replication and refinement. *Nursing Research, 37,* 240–244.

Gregor, F. (1981). Teaching the patient with ischemic heart disease: A systemic systematic approach to instructional design. *Patient Counseling and Health Education, 2,* 57–62.

Grose, B., & Woods, S. (1981). Effects of mechanical ventilation and backrest upon pulmonary artery and pulmonary capillary wedge pressure measurements. *American Review of Respiratory Disease, 123,* (Part 2), 120.

Grose, B., Woods, S., & Laurent, D. (1981). Effect of backrest position on cardiac output measured by the thermodilution method in acutely ill patients. *Heart & Lung, 10,* 661–665.

Hathaway, D., & Geden, E. (1983). Energy expenditure during late exercise program. *Nursing Research, 32,* 147–150.

Helton, N., Gordon, S., & Nunnery, S. (1980). The correlation between sleep deprivation and the intensive care unit syndrome. *Heart & Lung, 9,* 464–468.

Hilbert, G. (1985). Spouse support in myocardial infarction patients compliance. *Nursing Research, 34,* 217–220.

Hoel, B. (1978). Some aspects of the clinical use of thermodilution in measuring cardiac output. *Scandinavian Journal of Clinical Laboratory Investigation, 38,* 383–388.

Holm, K., Fink, N., Chrisman, N., Reitz, N., & Ashley, W. (1985). The cardiac patient and exercise: A sociobehavioral analysis. *Heart & Lung, 14,* 586–593.

Jansen, J., Schreuder, J., & Bogaard, J. (1981). Thermodilution technique for measurement of cardiac output during artificial ventilation. *Journal of Applied Physiology, 51,* 584–591.

Johnson, C., & Cowan, M. (1986). Relationships between the prolonged QTc interval and ventricular fibrillation. *Heart & Lung, 15,* 141–150.

Johnson, J., Rice, B., Fuller, S., & Endress, M. (1978). Sensory information, instruction in a coping strategy, and recovery from surgery. *Research in Nursing & Health, 1,* 4–8.

Johnston, B. (1984). Exercise testing for patients after myocardial infarction and coronary bypass graft surgery: Emphasis on predischarge phase. *Heart & Lung, 13,* 18–27.

Johnston, B., Cantwell, J., Watt, E., & Fletcher, G. (1978). Sexual activity in exercising patients after myocardial infarction and revascularization. *Heart & Lung, 7,* 1026–1031.

Johnston, B., Watt, B., & Fletcher, G. (1981). Oxygen consumption in hemodynamic and electrocardiographic responses to bathing in recent post myocardial infarction patients. *Heart & Lung, 10,* 666–671.

Jordan-Marsh, M., & Neutra, R. (1985). Relationship of health locus of control to life style change programs. *Research in Nursing & Health, 8,* 3–11.

Jouve, R., Puddu, P., & Torresani, J. (1982). Bretylium tosylate induced stabilization of electrical systole duration in patients with acute myocardial infarction. *Heart & Lung, 11,* 399–405.

Kadota, L. (1986). Reproducibility of thermodilution cardiac output measurements. *Heart & Lung, 15,* 618–622.

Keating, D., Bolyard, K., Eichler, E., & Reed, J. (1986). Effect of sidelying positions on pulmonary artery pressures. *Heart & Lung, 15,* 611–617.

Kennedy, G., & Crawford, M. (1984). The effects of lateral positioning on measurement of pulmonary artery and pulmonary artery wedge pressures. *Heart & Lung, 13,* 155–158.

Kinney, M. (1984). The scientific basis for critical care nursing practice: 1972–1982. *Heart & Lung, 13,* 116–123.

Kinney, M. (1985). Trends in cardiovascular nursing research: 1972–1983. *Cardiovascular Nursing, 21,* 25–30.

Kirchhoff, K., Rebensen-Piano, M., & Patel, M. (1984). Mean arterial pressure readings: Variations with position and transducer level. *Nursing Research, 33,* 343–345.

Kleven, M. (1984). Effect of backrest position on thermodilution cardiac output in critically ill patients receiving mechanical ventilation with positive end-expiratory pressure. *Heart & Lung, 13,* 303–304.

Kohanna, F., & Cunningham, J. (1977). Monitoring of cardiac output by thermodilution after open-heart surgery. *Journal of Thoracic and Cardiovascular Surgery, 73,* 451–457.

Larson, J., McNaughton, M., Kennedy, J., & Mansfield, L. (1980). Heart rate and blood pressure responses to sexual activity and a stair climbing test. *Heart & Lung, 9,* 1025–1030.

Laulive, J. (1982). Pulmonary artery pressures and position changes in the critically ill adult. *Dimensions of Critical Care Nursing, 1,* 28–34.

Lerman, J., Bruce, R., Sivarajan, E., Pettet, G., & Trimble, S. (1976). Low level dynamic exercises for earlier cardiac rehabilitation: Aerobic and hemodynamic responses. *Archives of Physical Medicine Rehabilitation, 57,* 355–360.

Levett, J., & Replogle, R. (1979). Thermodilution cardiac output: A critical analysis and review of literature. *Journal of Surgical Research, 27,* 393–404.

Lindsey, A. (1982). Phenomena and physiological variables of relevance to nursing, review of a decade of work: Part I. *Western Journal of Nursing Research, 4*, 343–364.

Lindsey, A. (1983). Phenomena and physiological variables of relevance to nursing, review of a decade of work: Part II. *Western Journal of Nursing Research, 5*, 41–63.

Lindsey, A. (1984). Research for clinical practice: Physiological phenomena. *Heart & Lung, 13*, 496–507.

Lindskog, B., & Sivarajan, E. (1982). A method of evaluation of activity and exercise in a controlled study of early cardiac rehabilitation. *Journal of Cardiac Rehabilitation, 2*, 156–164.

Manifold, S. (1984). A comparison of two alternative methods for the determination of cardiac output by thermodilution: Automatic vs. manual injection. *Heart & Lung, 13*, 304–305.

Mannesmann, G., & Muller, B. (1980). Measurement of cardiac output by thermodilution method in rats: The effect of different volumes and temperature of the indicator solution on cardiac output measurements and on cardiodynamics and hemodynamics of the anesthetized rat. *Journal of Pharmacological Methods, 4*, 11–18.

Mansfield, L., Sivarajan, E., & Bruce, R. (1978). Exercise testing of myocardial infarction patients prior to hospital discharge: A quantitative basis for exercise prescription. *Cardiac Rehabilitation, 8*, 17–20.

Marshall, J., Penckofer, S., & Llewellyn, J. (1986). Structured post operative teaching and knowledge and compliance of patients who had coronary artery bypass surgery. *Heart & Lung, 15*, 76–82.

McCance, K., Eutropius, L., Jacobs, M., & Williams, R. (1985). Preventing coronary artery disease in high risk families. *Research in Nursing & Health, 8*, 413–420.

Merrick, S., Hessel, E., & Dillard, D. (1980). Determination of cardiac output by thermodilution during hypothermia. *American Journal of Cardiology, 46*, 419–422.

Miller, P., & Shada, E. (1978). Preoperative information and recovery of open heart surgery patients. *Heart & Lung, 7*, 486–493.

Miller, P., Wikoff, R., McMahon, M., Garrett, M., & Johnson, N. (1982). Development of a health attitude scale. *Nursing Research, 31*, 132–136.

Mills, G., Barnes, R., Rodell, D., & Terry, L. (1985). An evaluation of an in-patient cardiac patient/family education program. *Heart & Lung, 14*, 400–406.

Minckley, E., Burrows, D., Ehrat, K., Harper, L., & Jenkins, S. (1979). Myocardial Infarct Stress of Transfer Inventory: Development of a research tool. *Nursing Research, 28*, 4–23.

Moodie, D., Feldt, R., & Kaye, M. (1979). Measurement of post-operative cardiac output by thermodilution in pediatrics and adult patients. *Journal of Thoracic and Cardiovascular Surgery, 78*, 796–798.

Murdaugh, C., & Hinshaw, A. (1986). Theoretical model testing to identify personality variables affecting preventive behaviors. *Nursing Research, 35*, 19–23.

Nakagawa-Kogan, H., Garber, A., Jarrett, M., Egan, K., & Hendershot, S. (1988). Self-management of hypertension, predictors of success in diastolic blood pressure reduction. *Research in Nursing & Health, 11*, 105–115.

Nelson, L., & Houtchens, B. (1982). Automatic vs. manual injections for thermodilution cardiac output determinations. *Critical Care Medicine,* *10,* 190–192.

Nemens, E., & Woods, S. (1982). Normal fluctuations in pulmonary artery and pulmonary capillary wedge pressures in acutely ill patients. *Heart & Lung, 11,* 393–398.

Nyamathi, A. (1987). The coping responses of female spouses of patients with myocardial infarction. *Heart & Lung, 16,* 86–92.

O'Connor, A. (1983). Factors related to the early phase of rehabilitation following aortocoronary bypass surgery. *Research in Nursing & Health,* *6,* 107–116.

O'Quinn, R., & Marini, J. (1983). Pulmonary artery occlusion pressure: Clinical physiology, measurement, and interpretation. *American Review of Respiratory Disease, 128,* 319–326.

Ott, C., Sivarajan, E., Newton, K., Almes, N., Bruce, R., Bergner, M., & Gilson, G. (1983). A controlled randomized study of early cardiac rehabilitation: The sickness impact profile as an assessment tool. *Heart & Lung, 12,* 162–170.

Pelletier, C. (1979). Cardiac output measurement by thermodilution. *Canadian Journal of Surgery, 22,* 347–350.

Penckoser, S. H., & Holm, K. (1984). Early appraisal of coronary revascularization on quality of life. *Nursing Research, 33,* 60–63.

Pender, N., & Pender, A. (1986). Attitudes, subjective norms and intentions to engage in health behaviors. *Nursing Research, 35,* 15–28.

Powner, D., & Snyder, J. (1978). In vitro comparison of six commercially available thermodilution cardiac output systems. *Medical Instruments,* *12,* 122–127.

Riedinger, M., & Shellock, F. (1984a). The effect of backrest elevation on pulmonary artery and pulmonary capillary wedge pressures in patients after cardiac surgery. *Heart & Lung, 13,* 691–692.

Riedinger, M., & Shellock, F. (1984b). Technical aspects of the thermodilution method for measuring cardiac output. *Heart & Lung, 13,* 215–222.

Riedinger, M., Shellock, F., & Swan, H. (1981). Reading pulmonary artery and pulmonary capillary wedge pressure waveforms with respiratory variations. *Heart & Lung, 10,* 675–678.

Rudy, E., Baun, M., Stone, K., & Turner, B. (1986). The relationship between endotracheal suctioning and changes in intracranial pressure: A review of the literature. *Heart & Lung, 15,* 488–494.

Runciman, W., Isley, A., & Roberts, J. (1981). An evaluation of thermodilution cardiac output measurement using the Swan-Ganz catheter. *Anaesthesiology Intensive Care, 9,* 208–220.

Sadler, P. (1981). Incidence, degree and duration of postcardiotomy delirium. *Heart & Lung, 10,* 1084–1092.

Schwartz, L., & Brenner, D. (1979). Critical care unit transfer: Reducing patients' stress through nursing interventions. *Heart & Lung, 8,* 540–546.

Shellock, F., & Riedinger, M. (1983). Reproducibility and accuracy of using room-temperature vs. ice-temperature injectate for thermodilution cardiac output determination. *Heart & Lung, 12,* 175–176.

Shellock, F., Riedinger, M., & Bateman, T. (1983). Thermodilution cardiac output determination in hypothermic post-cardiac surgery patients: Room vs. ice temperature injection. *Critical Care Medicine, 11,* 668–670.

Shinn, J., Woods, S., & Huseby, J. (1979). The effect of intermittent position pressure ventilation on pulmonary artery and pulmonary capillary wedge pressures in acutely ill patients. *Heart & Lung, 8*, 322–327.

Sivarajan, E., & Bruce, R. (1981). Early exercise testing after myocardial infarction. *Cardiovascular Nursing, 17*, 1–5.

Sivarajan, E., Bruce, R., Almes, N., Green, B., Belanger, L., Lindskog, B., Newton, K., & Mansfield, L. (1981). In hospital exercise after myocardial infarction does not improve treadmill performance. *The New England Journal of Medicine, 305*, 357–362.

Sivarajan, E., Lerman, J., Mansfield, L., & Bruce, R. (1977). Progressive ambulation in treadmill testing of patients with acute myocardial infarction during hospitalization: A feasibility study. *Archives of Physical Medicine Rehabilitation, 58*, 241–247.

Sivarajan, E., Newton, K., Almes, N., Kempf, T., Mansfield, L., & Bruce, R. (1983). Limited effects of outpatient teaching and counseling after myocardial infarction: A controlled study. *Heart & Lung, 12*, 65–73.

Skelley, B., Deeren, S., & Powaser, M. (1980). The effectiveness of two preoxygenation methods to prevent endotracheal suction induced hypoxemia. *Heart & Lung, 9*, 316–323.

Smyth, K., Hansell, S., Sparacino, J., & Strodbeck, F. (1978). Type A behavior pattern and hypertension among inner city black women. *Nursing Research, 27*, 30–35.

Snyder, J., & Powner, D. (1982). Effects of mechanical ventilation on the measurement of cardiac output by thermodilution. *Critical Care Medicine, 10*, 677.

Sparacino, J., Hansell, S., & Smyth, K. (1979). Type A (coronary prone) behavior and transient blood pressure change. *Nursing Research, 28*, 198–204.

Sparacino, J., Ronchi, D., Brenner, M., Kuhn, J., & Flesch, A. (1982). Psychological correlates of blood pressure: A closer examination of hostility, anxiety and engagement. *Nursing Research, 31*, 143–149.

Stawicki, J., Holford, F., & Michelson, E. (1979). Multiple cardiac output measurements in man: Evaluation of a new closed-system thermodilution method. *Chest, 76*, 193–197.

Steele, J., & Ruzicki, D. (1987). An evaluation of the effectiveness of cardiac teaching during hospitalization. *Heart & Lung, 16*, 306–311.

Stetz, C., Miller, R., & Kelly, G. (1982). Reliability of the thermodilution method in the determination of cardiac output in clinical practice. *American Review of Respiratory Disease, 126*, 1001–1004.

Swain, N., & Steckel, S. (1981). Influencing adherence among hypertensives. *Research in Nursing & Health, 4*, 213–222.

Swan, H., & Ganz, W. (1983). Hemodynamic measurements in clinical practice: A decade in review. *Journal of American College Cardiology, 1*, 103.

Tajiri, J., Katsuya, H., & Okamoto, K. (1984). The effects of respiratory cycle by mechanical ventilation on cardiac output measured using the thermodilution method. *Japanese Circulation Journal, 48*, 328–330.

Topf, M. (1984). A framework for research on aversive physical aspects of the environment. *Research in Nursing & Health, 7*, 35–42.

Toth, V. (1980). Effect of structured preparation for transfer on patient anxiety on leaving coronary care unit. *Nursing Research, 29*, 28–34.

Vanson, R., Katz, B., & Krekler, K. (1980). Stress effects on patients in critical care units from procedures performed on others. *Heart & Lung, 9,* 494–497.

Vennix, C., Nelson, D., & Pierpont, G. (1984). Thermodilution cardiac output in critically ill patients: Comparison of room-temperature and iced injectate. *Heart & Lung, 13,* 574–578.

Ventura, M., Young, D., Feldman, M., Pastore, P., Pikula, S., & Yates, N. (1984). Effectiveness of health promotion interventions. *Nursing Research, 33,* 162–167.

Weil, M. (1977). Measurement of cardiac output. *Critical Care Medicine, 5,* 117–119.

Whitman, C. (1982). Comparison of pulmonary artery catheter measurements in 20 degree supine and 20 degree right and left lateral recumbent positions. *Proceedings of the AACN International Intensive Care Nursing Conference, 120.* Newport, CA: American Association of Critical-Care Nurses.

Whitman, G., Howaniak, D., & Verga, T. (1982). Comparison of cardiac output measurements in 20-degree supine and 20-degree right and left lateral recumbent positions. *Heart & Lung, 11,* 256–257.

Wild, L. (1984). Effect of lateral recumbent positions on the measurement of pulmonary artery and pulmonary artery wedge pressures in critically ill adults. *Heart & Lung, 13,* 305.

Winslow, E., Lane, L., & Gaffney, F. (1985). Oxygen uptake in cardiovascular responses in control adults and acute myocardial infarction patients during bathing. *Nursing Research, 34,* 164–169.

Woodburne, T., & Powaser, M. (1980). Mechanisms responsible for the sustained fall in arterial oxygen tension after endotracheal suctioning in dogs. *Nursing Research, 29,* 312–316.

Woods, S., Grose, B., & Laurent-Bopp, D. (1982). Effect of backrest position on pulmonary artery pressures in critically ill patients. *Cardiovascular Nursing, 18,* 19–24.

Woods, S., & Mansfield, L. (1976). Effect of patient position upon the pulmonary artery and pulmonary capillary wedge pressure in non-acutely ill patients. *Heart & Lung, 5,* 89–90.

Woog, R., & McWilliam, D. (1983). A comparison of methods of cardiac output measurements. *Anesthesiology Intensive Care, 11,* 141–146.

Chapter 2

Prevention of Pressure Sores

CAROLYN E. CARLSON
DEPARTMENT OF NURSING
CEDARVILLE COLLEGE
CEDARVILLE, OH AND
REHABILITATION INSTITUTE OF CHICAGO
ROSEMARIE B. KING
REHABILITATION INSTITUTE OF CHICAGO

CONTENTS

The focus of this critical review is pressure sores. The chapter includes research on etiology, prediction, and prevention of pressure sores.

A pressure sore is defined as an area of soft-tissue damage, usually over a bony prominence, resulting from pressure of magnitude and duration sufficient to cause cell death. Pressure sores range from a superficial wound with erythema, induration, or ulceration (Grade 1) to severe necrosis of all soft tissues with bone involvement (Grade 4), according to Shea's (1975) system of classification.

MEDLINE and *Psychological Abstracts* searches were done using the key words *decubitus ulcers* (pressure sore and related terms), *prevention*, and *nursing* for the years 1967 through 1987. The *Cumulative Index to Nursing and Allied Health Literature* also was searched from 1982 through 1987. Reference lists from articles reviewed were another source of relevant literature. Although the major focus of this review was prevention of pressure sores, findings of earlier classic studies that contributed to the foundation for clinical investigations also have been summarized. In the brief description of early work an attempt has been made to point out contradictions in findings and threats to validity that rarely are mentioned in current literature. Only reports that included data based on systematic investigation of one or more variables associated with the development or prevention of pressure sores were reviewed.

FACTORS RELATED TO THE DEVELOPMENT OF PRESSURE SORES

The search for answers to the etiology of pressure sores has involved characteristics of the person and of the environment. Braden and Bergstrom (1987) have developed a conceptual schema with *pressure* and *tissue tolerance* as the primary concepts. Mobility, activity, and sensory perception influence pressure, whereas tissue tolerance is influenced by extrinsic factors (moisture, friction, shear) and intrinsic factors (nutrition, age, arteriolar pressure, and others). In addition to these factors, characteristics of the support surface and psychosocial environment are included in the review.

Environmental Factors

Physical and interpersonal environments can influence development of pressure sores. Pressure is the primary physical factor implicated in pressure sore development. Characteristics of the surface in contact with the skin are obvious factors to study; however, others include ambient temperature, humidity, and social–environmental factors such as availability of caregivers and care provided.

Contact Interface Variables. The response of soft tissues to pressure from external surfaces or objects has been the subject of much investigation. The widely cited work of Lewis and Grant (1925) indicated that reactive hyperemia, a protective response to pressure and an early sign of tissue damage, varied with pressure intensity and duration in two persons; it persisted for one half to three quarters of pressure duration. Data on duration of exposure to pressure were not provided. Kosiak (1959) also reported that hyperemia persisted half as long as pressure application. Later, using thermography to detect temperature in response to pressure in healthy subjects, Trandel, Lewis, and Verhonick (1975) reported that thermal flare persisted long after visual hyperemia in some subjects.

Landis's (1930) study of human skin capillary pressure established normal capillary pressure as 32 mm Hg, arteriolar; this value has been used as the threshold for tissue ischemia. More recently, Holstein, Nielsen, and Barras (1979) demonstrated that pressures approximating diastolic pressure were necessary to occlude skin circulation. Those data supported a threshold above 32 mm Hg to prevent tissue ischemia in most individuals. Using animal subjects, investigators demonstrated that tissue damage sometimes did not accompany pressures above capillary pressure applied for extended periods (Daniel, Priest, & Wheatley, 1981; Groth, 1942; Husain, 1953; Kosiak, 1959).

Research findings on intensity and duration of pressure have been basic to pressure sore prevention. Brooks and Duncan (1940) found duration of pressure more important in the etiology of pressure sores than intensity when pressures were at levels sufficient to produce tissue damage. Findings of a study of pressure-induced muscle necrosis in rabbits (Groth, 1942) included: (a) an inverse relationship between pressure intensity and duration necessary to produce a pressure sore; and (b) the most severe damage occurring in deep muscle. The findings on depth and severity of tissue damage were supported by Husain (1953) and Daniel et al. (1981).

Husain (1953) demonstrated that evenly distributed pressure created less damage than localized pressure and that moderate prolonged pressures resulted in more damage than intense pressure for short times. Kosiak's (1959) work supported Groth's (1942) finding of an inverse relationship between duration and intensity of pressure and of tissue damage. Contrary to the findings of Groth (1942), Husain (1953), and Daniel et al. (1981), Kosiak observed that tissue damage seemed to occur at all levels simultaneously. In another animal study, tissue damage was less following intermittent pressure than following constant pressure (Kosiak, 1961). Variations in subjects and techniques used and small numbers may have accounted for differences in findings. More study is needed to determine relationships between pressure intensity, duration, and tissue damage.

Bennett, Kavner, Lee, and Trainor (1979) measured shear, pressure, and local blood flow simultaneously to evaluate the effects of pressure and shear on circulation. The authors cited limitations of the instrument used, yet in all four subjects there was a trend toward occlusion at a lower pressure value in the high shear mode. Bennett, Kavner, Lee, Trainor, and Lewis (1981) measured skin blood flow in the seated position in 14 hospitalized older male patients (aged 67 and older) and 9 healthy younger men. Geriatric patients were more likely to experience greater shear values and blood flow occlusion at lower pressures. In another study, Bennett, Kavner, Lee, Trainor, and Lewis (1984) reported that shear values in healthy young men were approximately one third of those of geriatric and paraplegic subjects.

Dinsdale (1974) evaluated the effects of pressure and friction on the development of pressure sores in normal and paraplegic swine. Application of friction in addition to pressure was found to be a statistically significant factor in pressure sore development.

Brattgard, Carlsoo, and Severinsson (1975) provided evidence that wheelchair seats and covers resulted in a high temperature and humidity in the seat area. Environmental room temperature had a significant influence on sitting area humidity. In a study of 10 subjects with spinal cord injury and 10 normal subjects, Seymour and Lacefield (1985) reported no significant differences in skin temperature using eight wheelchair cushions. Number of subjects and other details were not discussed. Patterson and Fisher (1980) found in 12 persons with spinal cord injury that the temperature at the contact point between buttock and cushion decreased rapidly with wheelchair pushups.

Interpersonal Environment.   The interpersonal environment, including caregivers and providers of social support, has had potential for affecting pressure sore development; however, few investigators have included this variable. Lamid and El Ghatit (1983) reported that availability of help with skin care was unrelated to pressure sores. Anderson and Andberg (1979) found that patients with quadriplegia and paraplegia who were independent in skin care had lower pressure sore history scores than their counterparts with help in skin care. The relationships between help, responsibility, and satisfaction with activities need further study.

Person Factors

Williams (1972) conducted a multivariate study of 23 independent variables in newly hospitalized, nonambulatory patients to identify those factors associated with pressure sores. Although 147 subjects entered the study, data from only 26 could be used. Correlational and stepwise multiple regression analyses revealed age (younger), sex (males), body weight (thin), infection, body temperature, and corticosteroids to be related significantly to the development of pressure sores. Although sample size severely limits usefulness of the findings, the results provided evidence to support further study.

Demographic Variables. Age has been included in a number of investigations of etiology and incidence of pressure sores. Evidence of pressure sore incidence increasing with age has been reported in studies of hospitalized patients (Andersen & Kvorning, 1982; Bergstrom, Braden, Laguzza, & Holman, 1987a; Ek & Bowman, 1982; Manley, 1978; Pajk, Craven, Cameron-Barry, Shipps, & Bennum, 1986). A 24% incidence was reported among geriatric patients (Norton, McLaren, & Exton-Smith, 1962). Other studies of patients in extended care facilities (Gosnell, 1973) and of patients in adult units showed no relationship between age and pressure sores (Bergstrom, Demuth, & Braden, 1987b; Stotts, 1987). Williams (1972) reported a lower age group having more pressure sores, theorizing that it was probably an artifact of small sample size. Understanding of age and pressure sore relationships has remained incomplete because of methodological issues such as missing data (Versluysen, 1985), absence of control group or information about persons who did not develop sores (Anderson & Kvorning, 1982; Versluysen, 1985), lack of variance in age (Anderson & Kvorning, 1982; Gosnell, 1973; Norton et al., 1962; Versluysen, 1985), small sample size (Gosnell, 1973), absence or inadequate reporting of significance tests (Anderson & Kvorning, 1982; Gosnell, 1973; Versluysen, 1985), and inconsistent methods of assessing pressure sores.

Other demographic variables such as gender and education have been studied. Lamid and El Ghatit (1983) found no association between employment, education, caregiver presence, and independence and pressure sores. Cull and Smith (1973) reported no significant relationship between pressure sores and education or race in a study of patients with spinal cord injury. Significantly fewer pressure sores were reported among women. Details were not provided about pressure sore measurement or data collection. Ek and Bowman (1982) reported more pressure sores in women; however, they were overrepresented in the sample.

Anatomical and Physiological Variables. Body weight has been studied, but as a crude measure because factors that affect ideal weight such as height, age, and sex were not considered. Bergstrom et al. (1987b) reported that body weight of patients with pressure sores in intensive care, although less, was not significantly different from weight of subjects without pressure sores. Lamid and El Ghatit (1983) found no significant relationship between weight and pressure sores in a group of 38 patients with spinal cord injury.

Trandel et al. (1975) reported that maximum sacral pressure related poorly to height and weight but was related to size, shape, and topography of underlying bone as shown on thermography. No statistical tests were described.

Garber and Krouskop (1982, 1984) reported conflicting findings on the relationship between body build and seated pressures in patients with spinal cord injury. In the 1982 study, a significant relationship was found between thin body build and greater seated pressures. In an experiment (Garber & Krouskop, 1984) to determine the effectiveness of cushion modification on seated pressures, no significant relationships were found between pressures with modified or unmodified cushions and body build, sex, and level of injury.

In a study of relationships between blood flow and other variables in 29 healthy and 34 unhealthy adults, Ek, Lewis, Zetterqvist, and Svensson (1984) measured blood flow after heating the skin. Healthy persons under age 60 had greater blood flow response to heat over the hip than hospitalized subjects over age 60. Absence of details about methods and reliability of measures, uneven groups, and format of presentation have made evaluation and replication difficult. Seiler and Stahelin (1979) reported a linear decrease in oxygen tension with increasing pressure in healthy subjects. Bennett et al. (1984) reported similar median seated pressures (52 to 60 mm Hg) for subjects who were paraplegic ($n = 16$), hospitalized geriatric ($n = 14$), and normal ($n = 9$), with greatest variation in the paraplegic group. Using a reliable measure, median pulsatile blood flow was three times higher for the normals compared to the paraplegic and geriatric groups.

Gosnell's (1973) risk assessment study provided evidence that low diastolic pressure may be related to pressure sore development. All four patients who developed pressure sores had pressures under 60 mm Hg.

In practice, pressure tolerance is the length of time that an individual can be in one position with hyperemia resolving within a set time. Little research has been reported on tolerance variables such as acceptable duration of hyperemic response, individual differences, influencing factors, and the process of increasing tolerance.

A study of skin tolerance for pressure was conducted by Trumble (1930) using two subjects. The subject with lower blood pressure tolerated less pressure as measured by discomfort. The investigator suggested that skin pressure tolerance may vary with blood pressure values.

In studies involving continuous monitoring of pressure relief behavior of individuals with paralysis, intervals between pressure reliefs frequently exceeded the recommended intervals without development of pressure sores (Fisher & Patterson, 1983; Merbitz, King, Bleiberg, & Grip, 1985; Patterson & Fisher, 1980). Differences in time or unspecified time since injury, lack of information on reliability of measurement of pressure sores, and small and heterogeneous samples were limitations. The use of the microcomputer to provide continuous measurement of behavioral cues and responses (e.g., pressure reliefs) and the use of single-subject design (Merbitz et al., 1985) facilitated identification of pressure tolerance differences and effectiveness of preventive interventions.

Lifestyle/Psychosocial Variables.   Habits and psychological characteristics have had potential to exert at least indirect influence on tissue condition. Smoking has been investigated as a variable with potential for influencing pressure sore development (Lamid & El Ghatit, 1983) or severity (Lloyd & Baker, 1986). Both studies were of patients with spinal cord injury and involved multiple variables. In Lloyd and Baker's retrospective study of 60 inpatients with pressure sores, no association was found between location and severity of sores and smoking; the smoking classification was smoker or nonsmoker. In Lamid and El Ghatit's study, smoking, measured in pack years (packs per day times years smoked), was correlated significantly with incidence and severity of pressure sores.

Anderson and Andberg (1979) examined the relationship of several psychosocial variables and level of injury to pressure sores after discharge in 141 persons with spinal cord injury. Life activity satisfaction and responsibility for care were associated significantly with fewer days lost from activity (the measure of pressure sore incidence); however, reliability and validity of measures of responsibility and satisfaction were not described.

In a retrospective study, Gordon, Harasymiw, Bellile, Lehman, and Sherman (1982) investigated the association of hospital-acquired pressure sores with postrehabilitation psychosocial adjustment in 566 individuals with spinal cord injury. Reliability of pressure sore classification was questionable, and the method of data collection was not stated. Contrary to most studies of psychosocial variables, hospital-acquired pressure sores were viewed as a predictor of need for psychosocial services. The rationale for this suggested relationship so long after acute care was weak. As hypothesized, pressure sores were associated negatively with one adjustment subscale.

Participation in competitive sports and health maintenance was investigated by K. M. Stotts (1986) in individuals with paraplegia. Twenty-one athletes and 21 nonathletes completed questionnaires on demographic data and health. A friend or relative confirmed self-report. Groups were similar on several variables including preinjury involvement in sports. Significantly more pressure sores and more frequent hospitalizations were reported by nonathletes.

Illness/Disability Factors

Ek and Bowman (1982) reported on illness-related characteristics of 71 patients with pressure sores on 66 hospital wards. Thirty were immobilized; 52 were incontinent, and 30 had neurological disorders. Other investigators have reported on these variables.

Mobility.   Mobility was investigated by Exton-Smith and Sherwin (1961), who studied frequency of movement at night of 50 hospitalized elderly patients. Patients with less movement tended to develop sores. Although reliability and validity of the measures were not addressed, support was added to the importance of pressure relief. Manley (1978) reported that the greatest number of patients with pressure sores were partially helpless ($N = 30$). Lowthian (1979) found that 13 of 186 orthopedic patients had pressure sores. Of these, four were bedfast and four were chairfast. Contributing factors cannot be determined because so few had sores and the study was not longitudinal. Barbenel, Ferguson-Pell, and Kennedy (1986) measured overnight mobility of 40 hospitalized patients assessed for risk. High-risk patients moved less than the low-risk group. Sedation significantly reduced movements for both groups.

Incontinence and Fever.   Incontinence has been a common variable in risk scales used to predict pressure sore vulnerability. In a survey of incidence and factors contributing to pressure sore development, Manley (1978) found that all patients who were incontinent ($N = 28$) had pressure sores. In Gosnell's study (1973) incontinence was not a significant variable, but all four patients who developed pressure sores were febrile. Williams (1972) reported that elevated temperature and infection were associated with pressure sores but that incontinence was not related. In a study to identify age-specific characteristics on admission of 67 consecutive patients who developed pressure sores, N. A. Stotts (1987) reported that 45% had abnormal white blood counts.

Neurological Conditions. Neurological conditions that decreased sensation, mobility, and other functions have influenced pressure sore risk. Individuals with spinal cord injury have been vulnerable to pressure sores (Young & Burns, 1981). Anderson and Andberg (1979) reported evidence of greater severity of pressure sores in the paraplegic group than the quadriplegic group, despite similar incidence of pressure sores. Cull and Smith (1973) and Lamid and El Ghatit (1983) also reported no significant difference between level of injury and incidence of pressure sores; however, severity was excluded in the former and not significantly different in the latter.

METHODS OF PREVENTION

Based on literature on etiology of pressure sores, preventive strategies have included assessment and prediction of risk of pressure sores. Prevention has been attempted through use of surfaces to reduce pressure, changing position to reduce pressure, and education.

Assessment and Prediction Methods

An ideal measure of risk will be both sensitive and specific. Sensitivity is the percentage of persons predicted to develop pressure sores who actually developed sores, whereas specificity is the percentage of individuals who did not develop pressure sores and were not predicted to be at risk (Lilienfeld & Lilienfeld, 1980).

Norton Scale. The Norton Scale has been used in several prediction studies. Norton and colleagues (1962) described three investigations related to pressure sore prevention. In their study of etiological factors involved in the development of pressure sores, those investigators used a sample of 250 patients without pressure sores admitted to a geriatric unit. Five factors were assessed: (a) physical condition, (b) mental state, (c) activity, (d) mobility, and (e) incontinence. The mean Norton score at time of development of a pressure sore was 12.9, whereas the mean score for those without pressure sores was 15.7. Only skin breaks or blisters were considered pressure sores. Information was not provided on who rated the pressure sores or on the frequency of ratings. The vagueness of factors on the Norton Scale allows broad interpretation by the user. A similar limitation exists with the Gosnell (1973) scale.

Predictive validity of the Norton scale was investigated by Goldstone and Goldstone (1982) using 40 subjects matched on demographic and illness variables. Using a Norton score of 14 and under for predicting pressure sores, 89% of the subjects that developed lesions were in this category; however, 64% of those who did not develop sores also had scores of 14 or less. Groups differed significantly on Norton score.

A 5-factor scale derived from the Norton scale (Norton et al., 1962) was reported by Gosnell (1973). Multiple variables were assessed for 30 patients 68 years and older in four extended care facilities. Because of attrition, only 16 of the 30 patients were rated for the prescribed 4 weeks. None of the patients with low-risk scores developed pressure sores. Only four patients developed pressure sores; therefore, the sample size was too small to derive conclusions about the tool. Reliability of the scale, preventive nursing care provided, and pressure sore measurement were not described. The study findings were important in implicating blood pressure and elevated temperature in pressure sore development. Using the Gosnell Scale, Pajk and colleagues (1986) reported a significant association between lower mean risk score and pressure sores. Data provided in the latter study were insufficient to calculate sensitivity and specificity.

Andersen and Kvorning (1982) used a risk scale with seven variables including skin redness. Based on admission screening, 482 patients were assessed as at risk for pressure sores and 2,911 as not at risk. Reliability of ratings was not reported. Of those with no risk criteria, only five developed sores (.2%). Thirty-five of the patients at risk developed sores (5.8%). The scale was 87.5% sensitive and 86.6% specific. The authors observed that attention given to patients at risk may have influenced outcomes.

Braden Scale. The Braden Scale for Predicting Pressure Sore Risk consists of six subscales derived from the conceptual schema for the study of pressure sores described by Braden and Bergstrom

(1987). The subscales reflect the potential amount and duration of pressure and pressure tolerance (Bergstrom et al., 1987a, 1987b). The reliability of the scale has been investigated in three studies using registered nurse, licensed practical nurse, and nurse aide raters (Bergstrom et al., 1987a). Percent agreement is reported as 88% among nurse raters and 11% to 46% among other raters. The authors conclude that it is best to use nurse raters.

Three studies of predictive validity have demonstrated the sensitivity and specificity of predictions of pressure sores using various cutoff scores for prediction. In the first two studies implemented by Bergstrom, Braden and colleagues (1987), using a score of 16 or less, the Braden Scale was 100% sensitive and 90% specific in the first study ($N = 100$) and 100% sensitive and 64% specific in the second study ($N = 100$). In the third study involving 60 patients in intensive care (Bergstrom, Demuth, et al., 1987), the Braden Scale was 83% sensitive and 64% specific.

Thermography. Thermography was used by Newman and Davis (1981) to predict development of open areas in 91 patients on a geriatric unit. No patient with a normal thermogram developed a pressure sore within 10 days of admission. Six patients who developed pressure sores were among the 11 who had evidence of damage on admission thermography. The investigators compared predictions using thermography with predictions using the Norton Scale. Sensitivity (100%) and specificity (87%) were greater using thermography than using the Norton Scale (83% sensitivity and 63% specificity). Although this technique held promise for identifying occult tissue necrosis, the cost and inconvenience have prohibited its use.

In summary, several prediction methods have been developed to determine pressure sore risk. Comparisons of accuracy using specificity and sensitivity criteria provide evidence to support the Braden Scale as most promising (Table 2.1).

Preventive Interventions

Research on the effectiveness of preventive interventions such as patient education and control of risk factors has been limited.

Changing Position. The Conduct and Utilization of Research in Nursing (CURN) project (Horsley, Crane, Haller, & Bingle, 1981)

Table 2.1 Comparison of Specificity and Sensitivity Using Various
Methods to Predict Pressure Sore Development

Source	Method	N	Sensitivity	Specificity
Newman & Davis	Thermography	91	100%	87%
(1981)	Norton	88	83%	63%
Goldstone & Goldstone (1982)	Norton Scale	40	89%	36%
Bergstrom,	Braden	100	100%	90%
Braden, Laguzza, & Holman (1987a)	Braden	100	100%	64%
Bergstrom, Demuth, & Braden (1987b)	Braden	60	83%	64%
Gosnell (1973)*	Modified Norton	30	50%	73%

*Using a cut-off of 16.

included a two-part intervention based on Exton-Smith and Sherwin's (1961) study of spontaneous body movements and pressure
sores, and the finding that small shifts of body weight can allow for
hyperemia to occur under bony prominences (Miller & Sachs, 1974).
Risk assessment using the Norton Scale and unscheduled small shifts
of body position for patients at risk were the intervention activities.
Based on the CURN project, Brown, Boosinger, Black, and Gaspar
(1985) tested small body shifts. Fifteen patients who were in nursing
homes and rated at risk were assigned randomly to the experimental
(shifts and standard care) or control group (standard care only).
Despite greater risk in the experimental group, no patient developed
pressure sores, whereas one did in the control group. Data on later
risk scores were not included; therefore, assessment of the "Haw-
thorne effect" was not possible. The small number of subjects in
several facilities, lack of detail on measurement, and absence of
information on number of shifts were limitations.

Garber, Campion, and Krouskop (1982) measured pressures on
the trochanter when subjects with spinal cord injury were sidelying
with the upper leg in various positions. Extension of the upper leg
resulted in significantly less pressure in nondisabled persons and in
individuals with paralysis.

In a study of 100 female geriatric patients, Norton et al. (1962)
reported that frequent turning (every 2 to 3 hours) prevented pressure
sores in most cases. Procedural details such as reliability of turns,

controls, and statistical methods were not provided. Although this study provided evidence of effectiveness of regular repositioning, little research has been done on timing, type, and effectiveness of position change.

Teaching. Teaching programs have been developed to prevent pressure sores in patients at risk who are capable of performing preventive behaviors. Norris, Vise, Wharton, Noble, and Strickland (1982) tested the Spinal Injury Learning Series (SILS) using experimental and control groups at spinal cord injury system centers. Experimental and control groups were identified by center, with control groups receiving the usual respective center programs and the experimental groups using videotapes. The study findings were that the SILS produced faster acquisition, higher achievement, and longer retention of relevant knowledge and skills than the control groups after 1 year.

Another group of investigators (LaMantia et al., 1987) developed a multi-intervention preventive program for patients with chronic pressure sores. Twenty-eight persons with spinal cord injury (66% of those who started) completed the program. Of these, 24 (86%) remained healed 3 months later, and 15 of 23 (65%) continuing subjects remained healed at 1 year. Results that were analyzed statistically were impressive; however, the criteria for participation may have enhanced the probability of success. There was no control group, and the effectiveness of various aspects of the program was not stated.

Various devices and learning theory methods have been used to promote preventive skin care habits. Chawla, Andrews, and Bar (1978–1979) reported that patients became dependent on an automated reminder device. Malament, Dunn, and Davis (1975) used an avoidance conditioning program in which appropriate liftoff behavior avoided a negative stimulus. There was an effect on behavior in the two patients described; however, durability of pressure sore prevention behaviors was not reported. Use of automated and reminder devices has resulted in limited success (Klein & Fowler, 1981; Merbitz et al., 1985). Data based on larger numbers and long-term effectiveness are needed.

Using modeling, shaping, and social reinforcement to promote positioning behaviors, Rottkamp (1976) conducted an experimental study of 10 patients with spinal cord injury. The design provided limited control of intervening conditions affecting positioning and did not consider durability of behaviors.

Selecting Support Surfaces. Recent studies have been focused on the effects of various support surfaces on pressure reduction and pressure sore development. This review included all investigations of support surfaces by nurses identified in the search procedures as well as other studies that contributed important information about mattresses, beds, and cushions. Evidence has been provided that dynamic flotation surfaces can reduce pressure below capillary pressure (Redfern, Jenfid, Gillingham, & Lunn, 1973) and permit maintenance of high cutaneous PO_2 (Salisbury, 1985) for all bony sites tested. Other investigators have shown that various surfaces such as alternating pressure pads (Berjian, Douglas, Holyoke, Goodwin, & Priore, 1983; Krouskop, Williams, Krebs, Herszkowicz, & Garber, 1985), a static air mattress (Maklebust, Mondoux, & Sieggreen, 1986), a static dry flotation mattress and a foam-gel mattress (Krouskop et al., 1985), and a water bed (Wells & Geden, 1984) significantly reduced pressures compared to foam pads and standard mattresses. Berjian et al. (1983) concluded that a mud bed generally produced the lowest pressures when compared to seven surfaces. Investigators have shown trochanteric pressures to be greater than sacral pressure and frequently above capillary pressure (Krouskop et al., 1985; Maklebust et al., 1986), and approximately twice as high for ill patients compared to healthy subjects (Berjian et al., 1983).

Several researchers investigated effectiveness of various wheelchair cushions in reducing pressure, generally using persons with paralysis as subjects (Delateur, Berni, Hongladarom, & Giaconi, 1976; Garber, 1985; Mooney, Einbund, Rogers, & Stauffer, 1971). Mooney and colleagues (1971) reported the prefilled polyurethane cushion to be the best of 10 cushions tested by patients and controls, and Garber (1985) reported the static air cushion to be the best of 8 types in reducing pressure. DeLateur et al. (1976) investigated the duration of hyperemia in three patients using seven different cushions. None of the cushions prevented reactive hyperemia after motionless sitting for 30 minutes. No significant differences were found among the cushions.

Fisher, Szymke, Apte, and Kosiak (1978) investigated the effects of five cushions on skin temperature of healthy subjects and reported that the water cushion decreased temperature significantly. Bowker and Davidson (1979) studied healthy controls and 15 persons with disabilities to compare four cushions. A new gel cushion distributed pressure significantly better than all others.

Multiple problems exist in studies of support surfaces. Variability in the number and kind of support surfaces studied, lack of description of tests of significance (Berjian et al., 1983; Bowker & Davidson,

1979; Fisher et al., 1978; Garber, 1985; Mooney et al., 1971), and variations in subjects studied (e.g., healthy, disabled, ill) make comparisons difficult. Although variations in sidelying affect trochanteric pressure, several investigators did not report controlling for this variable (Berjian et al., 1983; Maklebust et al., 1986; Redfern et al., 1973). Despite the limitations, evidence supports the effectiveness of various surfaces in pressure reduction particularly for sacral pressures. Although dynamic flotation mattresses have reduced pressure below capillary pressure for all sites, no wheelchair cushion has reduced sitting pressures similarly.

In a clinical trial (Goldstone, Norris, O'Reilly, & White, 1982) patients with fractured femur were assigned alternately to a bead bed ($n = 32$) or to standard surfaces ($n = 43$). Groups were comparable in age and pressure sore risk. A significantly greater number of pressure sores developed using standard surfaces (48.8%) compared to experimental surfaces (16%). Skin assessment method and care were not described.

In a test of alternating air and silicone mattresses, Daechsel and Conine (1985) assigned 32 high-risk patients from long-term care facilities to study groups. Groups were comparable on demographic variables, weight, illness-related variables, and pressure sore risk rating. One investigator did skin assessments using the Exton-Smith rating scale. There was no significant difference in pressure sore incidence between groups over 3 months. Pressure relief frequency was not controlled.

Whitney, Fellows, and Larson (1984) investigated the relationships among risk factors, alternating pressure mattresses and foam overlays, and skin condition for 51 immobile patients. An adapted Norton Scale was used to assess risk. No reliability and validity data were provided for the scale or for measures of skin conditions. No variables were significantly associated ($p < .05$). Controlling for patient risk and initial skin condition, no difference was reported between groups using the two mattresses. The authors noted sample size, potential rater bias, and little variance in skin condition outcomes as weaknesses of the study. Control of pressure relief also was needed.

Ferguson-Pell, Wilkie, Reswick, and Barbenel (1980) followed 657 patients with spinal cord injury to demonstrate the importance of a pressure clinic in reducing ischial pressures. Results showed that there were significantly fewer sores in patients using cutout cushions designed to reduce pressure. Pressure relief activity was not known.

Despite missing details on procedure and limitations of the retrospective design, results provided evidence of the importance of pressure assessments when prescribing wheelchair cushions.

In a prospective controlled study, Hughes (1986) tested effectiveness of a flotation pad in prevention of sacral pressure sores in 100 patients over 75 years old, matched for age, with fractures of the femoral neck. The first 50 consecutive patients received standard care; the second group of 50 also used a flotation pad. A preliminary study of 40 patients with the same diagnosis showed that 35% developed a pressure sore. Analysis of the groups showed that 30% of control patients developed pressure sores, whereas only 2% of those using the flotation pad developed sores.

SUMMARY AND RECOMMENDATIONS

Much research has been done on the incidence, prevalence, etiology, and prevention of pressure sores. The work done represents multiple subject models and a variety of methods and settings. Generalizability and internal validity of findings of investigations are limited by the use of small or select samples (e.g., elderly, spinal cord injured), replication of only a few studies, and use of few comparison groups. In prediction and intervention studies, investigators frequently omitted describing preventive nursing care procedures that might have influenced outcomes.

Studies reviewed ranged from those with minimal control or detail about reliability and validity of procedure or analysis to carefully controlled experiments with explicit detail. Details on measurement methods were omitted frequently, and different methods were used to measure common variables, thus making comparisons of studies difficult. For example, classifications of pressure sores varied greatly among studies. In the research using pressure sore as outcome, investigators in 11 studies did not describe classification. Redness of unspecified duration or under 30 minutes was included as a Grade One pressure sore in six studies, whereas duration of hyperemia beyond 24 hours or persistent redness was used in three studies and blisters or broken skin were considered as Grade One in five studies. One study was difficult to classify. Variance in pressure sore classification may have accounted for some differences in findings.

Strengths in research on pressure sores include the use of advanced technology and the diversity in approaches. Variations in approaches are both strengths and weaknesses. The variations make comparisons difficult, yet they provide a useful foundation from which to build a model to demonstrate key relationships between variables that produce and prevent pressure sores. Common findings using different approaches strengthen the validity of study results.

Results provide evidence that numerous intrinsic and extrinsic variables may be implicated in pressure sore etiology. There is consistent support for pressure as a primary cause of soft tissue necrosis; however, findings on tolerance of pressure intensity and duration are inconsistent, and understanding of the role of friction, shear, and other mechanical factors is incomplete. Knowledge of conditions affecting tolerance could enable clinicians to alter external conditions and changeable intrinsic factors to increase pressure tolerance to a safe maximum time. Further study is recommended to determine changes in pressure tolerance over time and to determine the characteristics of persons who withstand pressures for durations that ordinarily would produce pressure sores. Age, mobility, elevated body temperature, and blood pressure variables have some support for contributing to etiology; however, few studies have been replicated.

Effective prediction instruments are promising in the prevention of pressure sores. Yet many questions remain unanswered about relationships between assessment scale, other variables, assessment methods, and interventions. For example, the state of knowledge about immobility does not enable clinicians to determine a pressure relief program matched to individual level of vulnerability. The role of psychological characteristics, social support, and other social-environmental variables in prevention essentially is unexplored.

Many pressure reduction surfaces are more effective than standard mattresses in reducing pressure. Evidence supports the use of dynamic flotation mattresses and selected static surfaces for high-risk patients. Few investigations have been focused on effectiveness of patient education and other preventive nursing interventions. To prevent pressure sores and to conserve resources, further studies are indicated to determine the effectiveness of visual hyperemia as an indicator of tissue damage; timed pressure relief (seated and recumbent); small body rotations; variations in positions; and interventions to control risk factors and promote self-care.

Technological advances make it possible to measure behavioral events and present cues in the absence of investigators. Devices can be used to assess the effects of planned or unplanned nursing interventions on pressure relief frequency (e.g., position changes, wheelchair reliefs) or the effects of training methods on behavioral compliance. The availability of reliable measures of pressure, pressure relief behavior, and stimulus behaviors improves the potential quality of research.

Knowledge can be expanded most effectively and efficiently if researchers develop more common approaches to assessment and measurement and view the problem of etiology and prevention of pressure sores as multivariate. The use of a conceptual model that includes demographic, physiological/pathophysiological, psychosocial, and physical–social–environmental variables as described in this review will facilitate development of comprehensive, systematic approaches to understanding pressure sore prevention.

REFERENCES

Andersen, K. E., & Kvorning, S. A. (1982). Medical aspects of the decubitus ulcer. *International Journal of Dermatology, 21*, 265–270.

Anderson, T. P., & Andberg, M. M. (1979). Psychosocial factors associated with pressure sores. *Archives of Physical Medicine and Rehabilitation, 60*, 341–346.

Barbenel, J. C., Ferguson-Pell, M. W., & Kennedy, R. (1986). Mobility of elderly patients in bed: Measurement and association with patient condition. *Journal of the American Geriatric Society, 34*, 633–636.

Bennett, L., Kavner, D., Lee, B. Y., & Trainor, F. A. (1979). Shear vs. pressure as causative factors in skin blood flow occlusion. *Archives of Physical Medicine and Rehabilitation, 60*, 309–314.

Bennett, L., Kavner, D., Lee, B. Y., Trainor, F. S., & Lewis, J. M. (1981). Skin blood flow in seated geriatric patients. *Archives of Physical Medicine and Rehabilitation, 62*, 392–398.

Bennett, L., Kavner, D., Lee, B. Y., Trainor, F. S., & Lewis, J. M. (1984). Skin stress and blood flow in sitting paraplegic patients. *Archives of Physical Medicine and Rehabilitation, 65*, 186–190.

Bergstrom, N., Braden, B. J., Laguzza, A., & Holman, V. (1987a). The Braden Scale for predicting pressure sore risk. *Nursing Research, 36*, 205–210.

Bergstrom, N., Demuth, P. J., & Braden, B. J. (1987b). A clinical trial of the Braden Scale for predicting pressure sore risk. *Nursing Clinics of North America, 22*, 417–428.

Berjian, R. A., Douglas, H. O., Holyoke, E. D., Goodwin, P. M., & Priore, R. L. (1983). Skin pressure measurements on various mattress surfaces in cancer patients. *American Journal of Physical Medicine, 62*, 217–226.

Bowker, P., & Davidson, L. M. (1979). Development of a cushion to prevent ischial pressure sores. *British Medical Journal, 2*, 958–961.

Braden, B., & Bergstrom, N. (1987). A conceptual schema for the study of the etiology of pressure sores. *Rehabilitation Nursing, 12*, 8–12.

Brattgard, S. O., Carlsoo, S., & Severinsson, K. (1975). Temperature and humidity in the sitting area. In R. M. Kennedi & J. M. Cowden (Eds.), *Bedsore biomechanics* (pp. 185–188). Baltimore: University Park Press.

Brooks, B., & Duncan, G. W. (1940). Effects of pressure on tissues. *Archives of Surgery, 40*, 696–709.

Brown, M. M., Boosinger, J., Black, J., & Gaspar, T. (1985). Nursing innovation for prevention of decubitus ulcers in longterm care facilities. *Plastic Surgical Nursing, 5*(2), 57–64.

Chawla, J. C., Andrews, B., & Bar, C. (1978–79). Using warning devices to improve pressure-relief training. *Paraplegia, 16*, 413–419.

Cull, J. G., & Smith, O. H. (1973). A preliminary note on demographic and personality correlates of decubitus ulcer incidence. *Journal of Psychology, 85*, 225–227.

Daechsel, D., & Conine, T. A. (1985). Special mattresses: Effectiveness in preventing decubitus ulcers in chronic neurologic patients. *Archives of Physical Medicine and Rehabilitation, 66*, 246–248.

Daniel, R. K., Priest, D. L., & Wheatley, D. C. (1981). Etiologic factors in pressure sores: An experimental model. *Archives of Physical Medicine and Rehabilitation, 62*, 492–498.

Delateur, B., Berni, R., Hongladarom, T., & Giaconi, R. (1976). Wheelchair cushions to prevent pressure sores: An evaluation. *Archives of Physical Medicine and Rehabilitation, 57*, 129–135.

Dinsdale, S. M. (1974). Decubitus ulcers, role of pressure and friction in causation. *Archives of Physical Medicine and Rehabilitation, 55*, 147–152.

Ek, A., & Bowman, G. (1982). A descriptive study of pressure sores: The prevalence of pressure sores and the characteristics of patients. *Journal of Advanced Nursing, 7*, 51–57.

Ek, A., Lewis, D. H., Zetterqvist, H., & Svensson, P. (1984). Skin blood flow in an area at risk for pressure sore. *Scandinavian Journal for Rehabilitation Medicine, 16*, 85–89.

Exton-Smith, A. N., & Sherwin, R. W. (1961). The prevention of pressure sores: The significance of spontaneous bodily movements. *Lancet, 2*, 1124–1126.

Ferguson-Pell, M. W., Wilkie, I. C., Reswick, J. B., & Barbenel, J. C. (1980). Pressure sore prevention for the wheelchair-bound spinal injury patient. *Paraplegia, 18*, 42–51.

Fisher, S., & Patterson, R. P. (1983). Long term pressure recording under the ischial tuberosities of tetraplegics. *Paraplegia, 21*, 99–106.

Fisher, S., Szymke, T. E., Apte, S. Y., & Kosiak, M. (1978). Wheelchair cushion effect on skin temperature. *Archives of Physical Medicine and Rehabilitation, 59*, 68–72.

Garber, S. L. (1985). Wheelchair cushions for spinal cord-injured individuals. *The American Journal of Occupational Therapy, 39*, 722–725.

Garber, S. L., Campion, L. T., & Krouskop, T. A. (1982). Trochanteric pressure in spinal cord injury. *Archives of Physical Medicine and Rehabilitation, 63*, 549–552.

Garber, S. L., & Krouskop, T. (1982). Body build and its relationship to pressure distribution in the seated wheelchair patient. *Archives of Physical Medicine and Rehabilitation, 63*, 17–20.

Garber, S. L., & Krouskop, T. (1984). Wheelchair cushion modification and its effect on pressure. *Archives of Physical Medicine and Rehabilitation, 65*, 579–583.

Goldstone, L. A., & Goldstone, J. (1982). The Norton score: An early warning of pressure sores? *Journal of Advanced Nursing, 7*, 419–426.

Goldstone, L. A., Norris, M., O'Reilly, M., & White, J. (1982). A clinical trial of a bead bed system for the prevention of pressure sores in elderly orthopaedic patients. *Journal of Advanced Nursing, 7*, 545–548.

Gordon, W. A., Harasymiw, S., Bellile, S., Lehman, L., & Sherman, B. (1982). The relationship between pressure sores and psychological adjustment in persons with spinal cord injury. *Rehabilitation Psychology, 27*, 185–191.

Gosnell, D. J. (1973). An assessment tool to identify pressure sores. *Nursing Research, 22*, 55–59.

Groth, K. E. (1942). Experimental studies on decubitus. *Nordic Medicine, 15*, 2423–2428.

Holstein, P., Nielsen, P. E., & Barras, J. (1979). Blood flow cessation at external pressure in the skin of normal human limbs. *Microvascular Research, 17*, 71–79.

Horsley, J. A., Crane, J., Haller, K. B., & Bingle, J. D. (1981). *Preventing decubitus ulcers CURN Project.* New York: Grune and Stratton.

Hughes, A. W. (1986). Prevention of pressure sores in patients with fractures of the femoral neck. *Injury, 17*(1), 19–22.

Husain, T. (1953). An experimental study of some pressure effects on tissues with reference to the bedsore problem. *Journal of Pathology and Bacteriology, 66*, 347–358.

Klein, R. M., & Fowler, R. S. (1981). Pressure relief training device: microcalculator. *Archives of Physical Medicine and Rehabilitation, 62*, 500–501.

Kosiak, M. (1959). Etiology and pathology of ischemic ulcers. *Archives of Physical Medicine and Rehabilitation, 40*, 62–68.

Kosiak, M. (1961). Etiology of decubitus ulcers. *Archives of Physical Medicine and Rehabilitation, 42*, 19–29.

Krouskop, T. A., Williams, R., Krebs, M., Herszkowicz, I., & Garber, S. (1985). Effectiveness of mattress overlays in reducing interface pressure during recumbency. *Journal of Rehabilitation Research and Development, 22*(3), 7–10.

LaMantia, J. G., Hirschwald, J. F., Goodman, C. L., Wooden, V. M., Delisser, D., & Staas, W. E. (1987). A program design to reduce chronic readmissions for pressure sores. *Rehabilitation Nursing, 12*(1), 2–25.

Lamid, S., & El Ghatit, A. Z. (1983). Smoking, spasticity and pressure sores in spinal cord injured patients. *American Journal of Physical Medicine, 62*, 300–306.

Landis, E. M. (1930). Micro-injection studies of capillary blood pressure in human skin. *Heart, 15*, 209–228.

Lewis, T., & Grant, R. T. (1925). Observations upon reactive hyperemia in man. *Heart, 12*, 73–120.

Lilienfeld, A. M., & Lilienfeld, D. E. (1980). *Foundations of epidemiology* (2nd ed.). New York: Oxford University Press.

Lloyd, E. E., & Baker, F. (1986). An examination of variables in spinal cord injury patients with pressure sores. *SCI Nursing, 3*(2), 19–22.

Lowthian, P. (1979). Pressure sore prevalence: A survey of sores in orthopedic patients. *Nursing Times, 72,* 358–360.

Maklebust, J., Mondoux, L., & Sieggreen, M. (1986). Pressure relief characteristics of various support surfaces used in prevention and treatment of pressure ulcers. *Journal of Enterostomal Therapy, 13,* 85–89.

Malament, J. B., Dunn, D. E., & Davis, R. (1975). Pressure sores: An operant conditioning approach to prevention. *Archives of Physical Medicine and Rehabilitation, 56,* 161–165.

Manley, M. T. (1978). Incidence, contributory factors, and costs of pressure sores. *South American Medical Journal, 53,* 217–222.

Merbitz, C. M., King, R. B., Bleiberg, J., & Grip, J. C. (1985). Wheelchair push-ups: Measuring pressure relief frequency. *Archives of Physical Medicine and Rehabilitation, 66,* 433–438.

Miller, M. E., & Sachs, M. L. (1974). *About bedsores.* Philadelphia: J. B. Lippincott.

Mooney, V., Einbund, M., Rogers, J., & Stauffer, E. (1971). Comparison of pressure distribution qualities in seat cushions. *Bulletin of Prosthetic Research, 10–15,* 129–143.

Newman, P., & Davis, N. H. (1981). Thermography as a predictor of sacral pressure sores. *Age & Aging, 10,* 14–18.

Norris, W. C., Vise, G. T., Wharton, G. W., Noble, C. E., & Strickland, S. B. (1982). The spinal cord injury learning series: An experimental test. *Archives of Physical Medicine and Rehabilitation, 63,* 243–247.

Norton, D., McLaren, R., & Exton-Smith, A. N. (1962). *An investigation of geriatric nursing problems in hospital.* London: The National Corporation for the Care of Old People.

Pajk, M., Craven, G. A., Cameron-Barry, J., Shipps, T., & Bennum, N. W. (1986). Investigating the problem of pressure sores. *Journal of Gerontological Nursing, 12*(7), 11–16.

Patterson, R. P., & Fisher, S. V. (1980). Pressure and temperature patterns under the ischial tuberosities. *Journal of Prosthetics Research, 17*(2), 5–11.

Redfern, S. J., Jenfid, P. A., Gillingham, M. E., & Lunn, H. F. (1973). Local pressures with ten types of patient-support system. *The Lancet, 2,* 277–280.

Rottkamp, B. C. (1976). A behavior modification approach to nursing therapeutics in body positioning of spinal cord injured patients. *Nursing Research, 25,* 181–186.

Salisbury, R. E. (1985). Transcutaneous PO_2 monitoring in bedridden burn patients: A physiological analysis of four methods to prevent pressure sores. In B. Y. Lee (Ed.), *Chronic ulcers of the skin* (pp. 189–195). New York: McGraw-Hill.

Seiler, W. O., & Stahelin, H. B. (1979). Skin oxygen tension as a function of imposed skin pressure: Implication for decubitus ulcer formation. *Journal of the American Geriatrics Society, 27,* 298–301.

Seymour, R., & Lacefield, W. (1985). Wheelchair cushion effect on pressure and skin temperature. *Archives of Physical Medicine and Rehabilitation, 66,* 103–108.

Shea, D. (1975). Pressure sores: Classification and management. *Clinical Orthopedics and Related Research, 112,* 89–100.

Stotts, K. M. (1986). Health maintenance: Paraplegic athletes and nonathletes. *Archives of Physical Medicine and Rehabilitation, 67,* 109–122.

Stotts, N. A. (1987). Age-specific characteristics of patients who develop pressure ulcers in the tertiary-care setting. *Nursing Clinics of North America, 22,* 391–398.

Trandel, R. S., Lewis, D. W., & Verhonick, P. J. (1975). Thermographical investigation of decubitus ulcers. *Bulletin of Prosthetics Research, 10,* 137–155.

Trumble, H. C. (1930). The skin tolerance for pressure and pressure sores. *Medical Journal of Australia, 17,* 724–726.

Versluysen, M. (1985). Pressure sores in elderly patients: The epidemiology related to hip operations. *Journal of Bone and Joint Surgery, 67*(1), 10–13.

Wells, P., & Geden, E. (1984). Paraplegic body-support pressure on convoluted foam, waterbed and standard mattress. *Research in Nursing and Health, 7,* 127–133.

Whitney, J. D., Fellows, B., & Larson, E. (1984). Do mattresses make a difference? *Journal of Gerontological Nursing, 10*(9), 20–25.

Williams, A. (1972). A study of factors contributing to skin breakdown. *Nursing Research, 21,* 238–243.

Young, J. S., & Burns, P. E. (1981). Pressure sores and the spinal cord injured: Part II. *SCI Digest, 3*(Winter), 11–26.

Chapter 3

The Effects of Stress During the Brain Growth Spurt

ELIZABETH M. BURNS
COLLEGE OF NURSING
THE OHIO STATE UNIVERSITY

CONTENTS

Special appreciation is extended to Thomas W. Kruckeberg of the College of Nursing, University of Iowa, and to Amy E. Shoemaker of the University of Iowa Hospitals and Clinics for their collaboration and assistance in the preparation of this chapter.

57

Behavioral Studies
Implications for Brain Development
Ethanol and Low Thyroxine During Ontogeny
Summary and Implications for Nursing Research

The developing brain, particularly during the brain growth spurt, responds to stressors (physical, chemical, environmental, nutritional, psychological, or social) differently from the adult brain. The difference in responsiveness is primarily because of the extremely rapid growth rate of the brain during the brain growth spurt. The human brain growth spurt extends from the beginning of the third trimester of pregnancy through the first two postnatal years. The rapidity of brain growth during this time frame is demonstrated by the fact that an infant's brain triples in size from birth to 2 years. In early postnatal life the infant's brain utilizes one half of its total caloric requirement to meet the nutritional and energy needs for the growth of its brain. The adult brain, on the other hand, uses only about one fifth of the total adult caloric requirement. Information relative to the potential dangers of stressors during the brain growth spurt is highly significant for nurses and other health care professionals involved in the care of mothers and infants. Research findings relevant to the effects of two selected stressors during the brain growth spurt are discussed in this chapter.

The brain growth spurt has been described as a "once only" opportunity for building the brain (Dobbing & Sands, 1971). The growth spurt is a period of maximal brain plasticity, a time when the brain is most capable of developing its genetic potential provided that the brain's environment is optimal. During the growth spurt the brain is critically sensitive and vulnerable to stressors such as a lack of nutrients or oxygen or the presence of harmful chemicals, any of which may lead to disruption of fundamental growth mechanisms.

Stress, defined as a stimulus, "is conceptualized as causing a disrupted response" (Lyon & Werner, 1987, p. 4). Stressors during the brain growth spurt may disrupt fundamental ontogenetic mechanisms; for example, membrane elaboration is a crucially important ontogenetic mechanism involved throughout embryological and fetal brain development. Disruption of membrane elaboration during synaptogenesis may interfere with (a) the development and outgrowth of axonal and dendritic growth-cones, (b) the outward movement of the leading edges of growth-cones resulting in the failure of axon terminals to find their targets, or (c) the recognition and adhesion processes that enable the establishment of synaptic connections. The resulting neuropathology is likely to affect neurological function and subsequently may be reflected in abnormal behavioral development.

CHEMICAL STRESS

Any chemical force capable of distorting or deforming brain cell membranes during any ontogenetic stage is a chemical stressor. During embryogenesis membrane deformation may affect cell proliferation, migration, or differentiation deleteriously and thus may lead to the development of gross neuropathology, observable at the light microscopic level or with the unaided eye. During the brain growth spurt, membrane deformation may disrupt the establishment of neuronal interconnections leading to fine structural pathology, detectable only at the electron microscopic level or by synaptic biochemical studies. Therefore, the presence of an unwanted chemical or the absence or deficiency of a needed chemical constitutes a chemical stressor that is either endogenous or exogenous depending on whether its origin is from within or outside the body.

Alcohol as an Exogenous Stressor

Alcohol is a timely example of an exogenous stressor because of its wide social use. Jones and Smith (1973) identified alcohol-induced birth defects as the fetal alcohol syndrome and attributed it to high maternal blood alcohol concentration during embryogenesis, as in alcoholism. A milder form of damage, fetal alcohol effects, is thought to be caused by exposure of the brain to low blood alcohol concentration, as in social drinking, during the brain growth spurt. Social use of alcohol in late pregnancy has been assumed to be innocuous. However, recent evidence suggests that this assumption is no longer tenable (Burns, Kruckeberg, Stibler, Cerven, & Borg, 1984; Stibler et al., 1983; Streissguth & LaDue, 1985).

Low Thyroxine as an Endogenous Stressor

During embryogenesis, thyroxine affects the mitotic machinery of brain cells, inducing cellular differentiation. Too little thyroxine interferes with the precise timing of messages to rapidly dividing cells to stop dividing and to begin migrating or myelinating. Too much thyroxine dramatically accelerates the tempo of neurophysiologic development, resulting in too many connections made too early (Ford & Cramer, 1977). Thus, abnormally low or high thyroxine levels constitute an endogenous chemical stressor. Investigators of the thyroxin dependency of locus coeruleus ontogeny (Seiger & Granholm, 1981) suggested that thyroxin is crucial for tubulin assembly, a process that is essential to the formation of neuronal processes. The tragic effects of untreated neonatal hypothyroidism highlight the importance of recognizing low thyroxine as an endogenous chemical stressor. The simultaneous presence of two stressors (low blood alcohol concentration and low thyroxine) undoubtedly would increase the risk of fetal brain damage.

THE FETAL ALCOHOL SYNDROME

The fetal alcohol syndrome is discussed here not because it develops during the brain growth spurt but so that relevant information about fetal alcohol syndrome may provide a backdrop against which fetal alcohol effects may be understood better. Of the two developmental problems, fetal alcohol syndrome is by far the more serious and is considered to be the major cause of mental retardation. It has not been reported except in the offspring of alcohol-dependent women. Because fetal alcohol syndrome neuropathology arises during the first 85 days of gestation, by the time it is recognized rehabilitation of the infant has been seriously compromised. Prevention, the only effective intervention, demands maternal abstention from alcohol throughout pregnancy. Although information concerning the etiology and consequences of fetal alcohol syndrome has been available for the past 15 years, prevention of this syndrome continues to be a challenge to health care professionals.

Much less is known about fetal alcohol effects. The synapse is thought to be the primary structure involved in its neuropathology.

The synapse provides the dynamic morphophysiological substrate for information processing, storage, and retrieval in the nervous system; therefore its integrity is essential to normal neurological function. Blood alcohol concentrations resulting from light or moderate social drinking are too low to cause the gross neuropathology of fetal alcohol syndrome during early pregnancy (Randall & Riley, 1984; Streissguth & LaDue, 1985) but, during the extremely vulnerable brain growth spurt, are sufficient to cause the fine structural neuropathology of fetal alcohol effects.

Women who are light or moderate social drinkers probably would abstain from alcoholic beverages during pregnancy and lactation if they were aware of the risk to fetal outcome. Recent clinical uses of alcohol for inhibition of premature labor, to increase the caloric content of solutions for hyperalimentation in premature infants, or as a solvent in pediatric medications have suggested that adequate information is not available concerning the possible harmful effects of low blood alcohol concentrations during brain ontogeny. Therefore, dissemination of information is essential to prevention of fetal alcohol effects.

Alcohol has been shown to be teratogenic in both experimental animals (Randall, 1977; Randall & Taylor, 1979) and in humans (Alpert et al., 1981; Clarren, Alvord, Sumi, Streissguth, & Smith, 1978; Clarren & Smith, 1978; Jones & Smith, 1973; Jones, Smith, Streissguth, & Myrianthopoulos, 1974; Landesman-Dwyer & Ragozin, 1981; Warren, 1977). Clinical studies have shown that the offspring of mothers whose daily alcohol intake is six drinks per day are at risk for fetal alcohol syndrome. What determines fetal susceptibility to the syndrome remains unknown [(Department of Health and Human Services (DHHS), 1987].

The constellation of developmental anomalies known as fetal alcohol syndrome includes: prenatal and postnatal growth deficiency; microcephaly; extensive neuropathology (neuroglial heterotopias, dysplasias, ectopic disorganized neuronal arrangements, and disruption of cell laminae and neuronal projections in the cerebral cortex, cerebellum and hippocampus); craniofacial dysmorphology; limb and organ anomalies; mental retardation (ranging from severe to moderate); and behavioral disorders.

The incidence of fetal alcohol syndrome is given as ranging from one to three per thousand live births in the total population and from 23 to 29 per thousand live births in infants born of a population including only alcoholic mothers (DHHS, 1987; Hanson, Streissguth,

& Smith, 1978). To date, the full-blown fetal alcohol syndrome has been observed only in offspring of chronically alcoholic women. Zinc deficiency is thought to contribute to the congenital abnormalities observed in fetal alcohol syndrome (Dreosti, 1984); however, this suggestion requires further research.

Etiology and Consequences

In the adult mammalian brain, alcohol and other solvents increase the fluidity of neuronal membranes, expand membrane surfaces, disorganize membrane constituents (i.e., alter lipid compositon, distort the stearic arrangement of proteins, and alter the carbohydrate composition of various membrane-bound glycoconjugates), affect the activity of membrane-bound enzymes, and disturb membrane transport mechanisms (Hunt, 1985). Alcohol also decreases the synthesis of brain nuclear and mitochondrial ribonucleic acid (RNA); adversely affects the proper association of ribosomal subunits, in turn affecting protein synthesis; inhibits the increase of glucose utilization that occurs in activated neurons; and inhibits $Na+/K+$ ATPase at high blood alcohol concentrations, in turn interfering with brain carbohydrate metabolism that is associated with increased brain glucose levels (Tabakoff, Noble, & Warren, 1979). Alcohol dissolves in neuronal membrane lipids. Because of the high lipid content of the synaptic portions of the neuronal membrane, the synapse is the prime target of the harmful effects of alcohol. Thus, it is not surprising that alcohol is detrimental to developing neuronal membranes.

Alcohol-induced undernutrition has been thought to play a role in fetal alcohol syndrome etiology. In extensive studies of nutritional factors Samson and Grant (1985), however, indicated that alcohol affects the brain directly. They proposed that the effects of alcohol are mediated by alcohol–membrane interactions, alcohol-induced changes in cellular metabolism, and alterations in cellular secretions. Further, Samson and Grant (1985) suggested that the direct effects of alcohol may be increased by a less than optimal nutritional status, a condition frequently associated with heavy alcohol intake.

Altered prostaglandin metabolism was proposed by Randall, Anton, and Becker (1987) as a biochemical molecular basis for the teratogenic effects of alcohol. However, they pointed out that the exact relationship between alcohol, pregnancy, and prostaglandins remains to be elucidated by future research.

Microcephaly, a key characteristic of fetal alcohol syndrome, probably results from the direct effect of alcohol on the brain, with subsequent accommodation of cranium size to brain size. Similarly, prenatal and postnatal growth deficiency may be due to the effect of alcohol on growth hormone production primarily, and only secondarily to an altered nutritional status. Growth depends on the availability of substrates that provide the components needed for cell growth and for production of hormones that regulate growth rate. Hall and Sara (1983) reported that somatomedins regulate fetal brain growth and that their neuromodulatory role is essential for the maintenance of mature brain cells. Preliminary studies of Sara and Tham (1985) gave evidence that maternal alcohol intake impairs not only maternal but also fetal somatomedin production. Maternal somatomedin levels correlate with fetal growth (Sara, Gennser, & Persson, 1982; Sara, Hall, Rodeck, & Wetterberg, 1981).

Specific brain regions, the hippocampus (Barnes & Walker, 1981; West & Hamre, 1985; West, Hodges, & Black, 1981) and the locus coeruleus (Strahlendorf & Strahlendorf, 1983), have been shown to be sensitive to alcohol selectively. Thus, damage to the developing hippocampus likely would compromise its future role in learning. Numerous functions have been proposed for the locus coeruleus, including normal and abnormal processes associated with memory, attention, reinforcement, anxiety, fear, sleep and arousal, motor control, dementia, depression, and schizophrenia (Mason, 1981; Van Dongen, 1981). Therefore, damage to the locus coeruleus during its ontogeny likely would compromise its future functional role. Much remains unknown about the actual mechanisms that mediate the expression of the characteristics of fetal alcohol syndrome. Further elucidation of the etiology of this syndrome demands continued research.

Diagnosis, Intervention, Prevention

Evidence of maternal alcoholism or alcohol abuse usually is considered essential for a diagnosis of fetal alcohol syndrome. Criteria for its diagnosis (Streissguth, 1986; Weiner & Larson, 1987) include the presence of three primary characteristics: (a) growth deficiency; (b) a cluster of facial abnormalities (short palpebral fissures, low nasal bridge, absent or indistinct philtrium, thin upper lip with a narrow vermilion border, short or upturned nose, epicanthal folds, and a flat midface); and (c) central nervous system damage. Malformations of the skeletal, urogenital, and cardiovascular systems also are observed frequently. Failure to thrive and a weak sucking reflex during the neonatal period have been observed (Van Dyke, Mackay, & Ziaylek, 1982). At birth infants with fetal alcohol syndrome may be tremulous, irritable, and hypersensitive to sound (Streissguth, 1986).

Immediate intervention in fetal alcohol syndrome is focused on the presenting symptoms. Failure to thrive, hypotonia, poor fine and gross movements, delayed development, and mental retardation are among the debilitating aspects that persist. Prevention includes two major components, dissemination of information and prenatal counseling. Research to date has indicated that a safe level of maternal alcohol intake is not known and that the only safe course for pregnant women is abstinence from prior to conception throughout lactation.

FETAL ALCOHOL EFFECTS

The severity of alcohol-induced brain deficits ranges from full-blown fetal alcohol syndrome to the more subtle though serious abnormalities described as fetal alcohol effects. The causative agent is the same in both, although there are differences in the timing, intensity, and duration of exposure to the agent. Fetal alcohol syndrome is attributed to chronic exposure during the first trimester or pregnancy to a high blood alcohol concentration, whereas fetal alcohol effects are attributed to briefer exposures during the brain growth spurt to low blood alcohol concentrations. Fetal alcohol effects include attention deficit disorder (Shaywitz, Griffieth, & Warshaw, 1979), hyperactivity (Clarren & Smith, 1978), and other less clearly understood brain deficits resulting from alcohol-induced fine structural neuropathology. Other contributory factors, however, may be involved.

Etiology and Consequences

Fetal alcohol effects neuropathology is primarily a result of the effects of alcohol on membranes during synaptogenesis. However, alcohol also depresses synaptic function (Fox et al., 1978; Lewis & Boylan, 1979; McLeod et al., 1983, 1984), thereby decreasing feedback to the synapse. Normal feedback is essential for maturation of the synapse (Burry, Kniss, & Scribner, 1984).

Because the human brain growth spurt is perinatal, including not only the third trimester of pregnancy but also the first two postnatal years, it is important to examine how the developing brain inadvertently may be exposed to significant blood alcohol concentrations.

Landesman-Dwyer (1981) reviewed the use of alcohol for inhibition of premature labor. Although selective beta-2 agonists were found to be useful for this purpose (Weiner, 1980), alcohol has continued to be used to some extent (Andersson, 1982; Caritis et al., 1982; Caritis, Edelstone, & Mueller-Heubach, 1979; Fuchs & Fuchs, 1981; Fuchs, Fuchs, Lauersen, & Zervoudakis, 1979; Souney, Kaul, & Osathanondh, 1983). Sisenwein, Tejani, Boxer, and DiGiuseppo (1983) reported that a subgroup of children born within 15 hours of alcohol infusion showed significant pathology on developmental testing and personality inventory at 4 to 7 years of age. Behavioral assessment of such children has been extremely limited (Landesman-Dwyer, 1981).

Alcohol also was used in hyperalimentation in small-for-date infants. Infantile intoxication during hyperalimentation was reported by Peden, Sammon, and Downey (1973), who found blood alcohol concentrations as high as 163 to 183 mg/dl in several lethargic premature infants. Cook, Shott, and Andrews (1975) stressed the dangers of alcohol in hyperalimentation solutions for premature infants.

Social drinking duration lactation is not without danger. The concentration of alcohol in human milk becomes measurable within 30 minutes after the ingestion of a drink, and a significant level persists for several hours (Kerfoot, Kruckeberg, & Burns, 1985; Kesaniemi, 1974). Alcohol 0.6 g/kg (15% solution in water) consumed in 5 minutes yielded a peak milk alcohol concentration of 78 mg/dl in 30 minutes (Kesaniemi, 1974), and alcohol 1 g/kg (10% solution in grapefruit juice) consumed slowly in 3 hours yielded a peak milk alcohol concentration of 90 mg/dl in 3 hours and 45 minutes (Kerfoot et al., 1985).

The American Academy of Pediatrics (AAP) (1984) Committee on Drugs found 700 liquid pediatric pharmaceutical preparations containing alcohol in concentrations ranging from .35 to 68%. The work of the American Academy of Pediatrics Committee influenced some (not all) pharmaceutical companies to remove alcohol from liquid pediatric medications.

Clearly, the human brain inadvertently can be exposed to low blood alcohol concentrations during the brain growth spurt. Because of the crucial vulnerability of the brain during this time frame, the resulting subtle, fine structural neuropathology at the molecular, biochemical level may have serious consequences for neurobehavioral development. Fetal alcohol effects are thought to be related causally to attention deficit disorder, hyperactivity, and other behavioral teratological disorders. Further research is needed to define more clearly the neuropathology and the mechanisms mediating fetal alcohol effects, as well as to design programs for rehabilitation of affected individuals.

Recently, Inomata, Nasu, and Tanaka (1987) found, in an animal model, an alcohol-induced decrease in the numerical density of synpases in the frontal cortex. They suggested that there may be a relationship between frontal cortex synaptic density and mental development, a suggestion that demands further research.

Diagnosis, Intervention, Prevention

Diagnostic criteria for fetal alcohol effects have not been delineated clearly but would include confirmation of maternal drinking pattern and/or infant's ingestion of alcohol via breast milk or liquid medications. Prevention is the primary effective intervention and includes dissemination of information to health professionals, to the clientele in the maternal-child health arena, and to the general public about the potential dangers of alcohol during the brain growth spurt. Prevention also should include counseling for optimal nutrition and exercise, general health promotion, and environmental enrichment, especially from a psychosocial viewpoint. Although the early postnatal period is a time of crucial vulnerability, it is likewise a time of maximal brain plasticity; therefore one can expect maximal responsiveness to early, aggressive rehabilitative efforts.

VULNERABLE PERIODS IN BRAIN DEVELOPMENT

An important teratological principle is: The more rapid the growth rate of a tissue, the greater is its vulnerability. Based on this principle, three phases of human neuro-ontogeny have been identified as critically vulnerable periods: (a) organogenesis (gestation weeks 3 to 9); (b) rapid neuronal proliferation (gestation weeks 12 to 20); and (c) the brain growth spurt (gestation weeks 30 to 40 and the first 18 to 24 months after birth).

In general, central nervous system development (in contrast to development of the rest of the organism) proceeds in a sequential caudocranial manner (Timiras, Vernadakis, & Sherwood, 1968), with maturation of the spinal cord preceding that of myelencephalon, mesencephalon, diencephalon, and telencephalon respectively (Vernadakis & Woodbury, 1969). For example, a major portion of cerebellar development occurs postnatally (Altman, 1969, 1972a, 1972b, 1972c; Ito, 1984; West, 1987). Thus, during any specific time frame, selective and significant exposure to teratogen may affect the specific brain region, system, or part of a system most vulnerable at the precise time of exposure.

Organogenesis

Organogenesis (gestation weeks 3 to 9) is a time of critical vulnerability for the entire organism. Neuro-ontogenetic events characteristic of this developmental phase include establishment of the basic embryonic plan of the brain and induction of the future central and peripheral nervous systems. These events are mediated by cell proliferation, migration, differentiation, and cellular death. The effects of teratogenic agents during organogenesis are likely to be devastating and may give rise to major deformities or embryonal death (Moore, 1977). In this light, a 17% perinatal mortality rate in offspring of alcoholic women as compared with 2% for nonalcoholic women (Jones et al., 1974) is not surprising. Further, Clarren and Smith (1978) observed gross neuropathology (neuroglial heterotopias, dysplasias, and ectopic disorganized neuronal arrangements) in the brains of infants who died perinatally and whose mothers were chronic alcoholics. These neuropathological changes probably resulted from injury during organogenesis (Lemire, Loeser, Leech, & Alvord, 1975). Dow and Riopelle (1985) have suggested that alcohol alters neuronal growth cone formation and the production of neurotrophic factors, thus interfering with essential mechanisms mediating embryonal central nervous system development.

Rapid Neuronal Proliferation

A second vulnerable period in human brain ontogeny (Dobbing, 1974) occurs during gestation weeks 12 to 20. No studies have been reported concerning the effects of alcohol during this period of rapid proliferation. The anticipated effect would be fewer brain cells.

The Brain Growth Spurt

The final critically vulnerable period for the developing human brain begins during the last trimester of pregnancy and continues throughout the first 18 to 24 months after birth. This time frame encompasses the most rapid phase of brain growth and is known as the brain growth spurt. It is characterized by dendritic arborization, axonal growth, peak synaptogenesis, gliogenesis, myelination, and maturation of structures and mechanisms involved in synaptic neurotransmission (Dobbing, 1971; Dobbing & Sands, 1979; Dobbing & Smart, 1973).

Because of the key role of the synapse in the maintenance of nervous system integrity, the effects of alcohol during the brain growth spurt on synaptic biochemical ontogeny are of particular interest. The synapse provides the dynamic physical substrate of interneuronal communication and information processing. Whatever affects the synapse will affect neurological function, cognition, and behavior. Synaptogenesis is the single most important event during brain development for achieving optimal, appropriate interneuronal connections. Some of the most obvious and frustrating effects of damage during this time frame are hyperkinesis, impaired learning, and behavioral problems in children. Damage during the brain growth spurt is likely to be permanent unless rehabilitation is undertaken soon after birth. The period of maximal synaptic plasticity, the time of greatest potential for optimal development, coincides with that of maximal synaptic vulnerability. If synaptic damage has occurred prior to birth, aggressive intervention during early postnatal life may repair the damage to some extent. If rehabilitation is delayed beyond the brain growth spurt, repair possibility is minimal.

Burry et al. (1984) recently hypothesized that synaptogenesis proceeds by a series of events in which completion of a preceding event is required before the subsequent event is initiated. Completion of the sequence of events in an orderly manner enables development of the synaptic machinery required for effective synaptic function.

Feedback from functional activity of the developing synapse is essential to synaptic maturation.

During ontogeny, terminals of axons must find and attach to their appropriate targets. This process involves guided outgrowth of the leading edge of the growth cone, recognition of appropriate target sites, and attachment and adhesion of presynaptic and postsynaptic elements. Four factors that influence the recognition-adhesion process are humoral substances, intercellular matrix, cell surfaces, and feedback. The single most important of these factors is the cell surface, that is, synaptic plasma membrane microarchitectonics or "signatures" on the leading edge of the growth cone and on the future postsynaptic target site. Numerous investigators have shown that alteration of these "signatures," that is, alteration of the biochemical molecular structure of the involved membranes, leads to changes in cellular behavior (Edelman, 1976, 1983, 1985; Rothbard, Brakenbury, Cunningham, & Edelman, 1982).

During synaptogenesis, alcohol-induced alterations in membrane fluidity known to occur in adult neuronal membranes would be expected to distort "signatures" of developing synaptic elements. If so, the sequential series of synaptic events would be disturbed and normal synaptogenesis disrupted. Also, alcohol depresses synaptic function, decreasing feedback to the synapse and further disturbing normal synaptogenesis. Further, alcohol probably would interfere simultaneously with blood–brain barrier ontogeny. Disruption of the blood–brain barrier then might subject the brain to other circulating toxins from which it otherwise would have been spared.

TERATOLOGICAL STUDIES DURING THE BRAIN GROWTH SPURT

Until recently, the concept of teratology was focused primarily on fetal morphological malformations that were observed either by the unaided eye or at the light microscopic level. These malformations frequently were gross and sometimes incompatible with life. This type of dysmorphology is demonstrable in infants who die perinatally because of full-blown fetal alcohol syndrome. Findings from electron microscopic and biochemical molecular studies have led to an expanded concept of teratology, focused on ultrastructural dysmorphology and related neurological dysfunction. The implications of synaptic dysmorphology for behavioral maldevelopment thus gave rise to a concept of behavioral teratology.

The Postnatal Rat as an Animal Model

The brain growth spurt in the rat is completely postnatal. The major portion of the peak of the brain growth spurt occurs during days 6 to 16 after birth. The neuro-ontogenetic events observed in the rat during days 1 to 10 after birth are comparable to those occurring in the human during the third trimester of pregnancy. The neuro-ontogenetic events observed in the rat during days 11 to 21 postnatally similarly are comparable to those occurring in the human during the first five or six months postnatally (Dobbing, 1971; Dobbing & Smart, 1973). Therefore, the preweanling rat serves as a useful model for pharmacological studies of the developing brain. This model enables the investigation of the direct effects of alcohol exposure during the brain growth spurt because alcohol can be administered to postnatal rats directly via gavage, thus avoiding confounding indirect effects. For example, if alcohol were administered to lactating rat dams and via the milk to rat pups, the indirect effects of alcohol would include its effects on maternal behavior, maternal nutritional status, and on lactation. All of these factors undoubtedly would confound the direct effects of alcohol on the developing brain.

Biochemical Studies

To test the hypothesis that chronic exposure to low blood alcohol concentrations during the brain growth spurt alters synaptic biochemistry and ultrastructure, Burns and colleagues (Burns et al., 1984; Stibler et al., 1983) administered alcohol 4 g/kg body weight via gastric gavage daily (in fractional doses) during the major portion of the peak of the rat brain growth spurt, that is, on postnatal days 6 through 16. The selected dose of alcohol, 4 g/kg body weight, is approximately one third of the dose used in the same animal model to mimic maternal alcoholism. The rate for the metabolism of alcohol in the rat is approximately three times as fast as that in the human; thus the 4 g/kg body weight dose in the rat would be comparable to moderate social drinking in the human.

The results revealed significantly reduced synaptosomal sialic acid content, significantly diminished activity of ecto-sialyltransferase, and no change in neuroaminidase activity. The sialic acid was distributed equally between glycoprotein-bound and glycolipid-bound sialic acid. No change was found in either the total protein or lipid content of synaptosomes (Stibler et al., 1983). Additional evidence from studies in litter mates of the animals used for the biochemical studies revealed no effect of alcohol 4 g/kg body weight on body temperature in preweanling rats (Kruckeberg et al., 1984). Thus, the altered synaptic biochemistry was not because of alcohol-induced hypothermia but rather the direct pharmacological effects of alcohol.

Sialic acid is thought to be a constituent of the "signatures" on growth cones and their target sites. Decreased synaptosomal sialic acid content could, therefore, interfere with normal synaptogenesis; this neuropathology then might be reflected in problems associated with fetal alcohol effects. Later, in another group of animals using the same treatment design, altered synaptosomal galactose content was found (Stibler, Burns, Kruckeberg, Cerven, & Borg, 1985); however, no difference in synaptosomal Na+/K+-ATPase activity was noted.

Ultrastructural Studies

Micromorphological studies in these animals revealed nonsignificant structural changes in the cerebellum, lobule IX, at the light and electron microscopic levels (Burns et al., 1984). The numbers of cerebellar Purkinje cells and synaptic profiles per unit volume were less in alcohol-treated than in control animals, but these differences were not statistically significant. Thus the subtle damage that was significant at the biochemical level was not statistically significant at the micromorphological level. However, the trends were consistent across all parameters. A decreased number of cerebellar cells (based on DNA content) was observed in alcohol-treated animals. Obviously, further studies are indicated.

Behavioral Studies

Preliminary studies of the effects of alcohol on balancing ability were performed using the same animal model. Burns, Kruckeberg, Kanak, and Stibler (1986) compared the effects of alcohol 6 g/kg on postnatal day 6 (as in episodic or binge drinking) with the effects of 4 g/kg on days 6 through 16. The 6 g dose in a rat is equivalent to approximately five drinks on one occasion. On days 17 and/or 70, animals were tested for their balancing abilities. All alcohol-treated animals performed less well than controls on three tests of balancing ability (balance beam, roto-rod, and inclined plane), but not at a statistically significant level (Burns et al., 1986).

Implications for Brain Development

Body, whole brain, and cerebellar weights were significantly lower in both groups of alcohol-treated rats as compared with controls on postnatal day 17. By 70 days of age no between-group body weight differences in either males or females were observed; however, between-group whole brain and cerebellar weight differences remained. At both 17 and 70 days after birth in the two alcohol-treated groups, the cerebellum was decreased disproportionately in weight with respect to the brain as a whole. The number of cerebellar cells (based on DNA content) also was decreased significantly in both sexes in the two alcohol-treated groups, as compared with controls.

These results underline the importance of timing, intensity, and duration of alcohol exposure during ontogeny and the lasting effects that can be produced during this critically vulnerable phase. Even within the time frame encompassed by the most rapid phase of brain growth as a whole, specific systems or parts of systems are growing more rapidly at one precise time than another (West, 1987); consequently, they are more vulnerable at their time of most rapid growth.

A proposed criterion of nutritional adequacy in animals treated with alcohol during ontogeny (Wiener, Shoemaker, Koda, & Bloom, 1981) is normalcy of body and brain weights. Dobbing and colleagues (Dobbing, 1971; Dobbing & Smart, 1973; Sands & Dobbing, 1981) found brain weight to be less affected than body weight by malnutrition, which gave rise to the misleading concept of "brain sparing." Although brain weight is affected less than body weight by malnutrition during the brain growth spurt, a small decrement localized to a critical area can be extremely important. For example, a critical decrease in numbers of neurons or synaptic connections within a small circumscribed brain region (e.g., the locus coeruleus, hippocampus, cerebellum, or brain stem nuclei) might affect neurological function seriously without significantly altering brain weight.

According to Dobbing and Sands (1971), an irreversible true microcephaly results in rats exposed to severe malnutrition during the brain growth spurt. Dobbing and Smart (1973) showed that retardation of body growth by malnutrition through the brain growth spurt also results in a permanent body weight deficit that resists rehabilitative efforts.

Microcephaly is the cardinal characteristic of fetal alcohol syndrome. The significantly decreased brain weights in alcohol-treated rats as compared with controls showed a trend toward microcephaly. Fetal alcohol syndrome is not thought to be produced by severe nutritional deprivation in the absence of alcoholism per se; thus, microcephaly is a direct pharmacological effect of alcohol, with subsequent accommodation of the infant's head size to its small brain size. Therefore, the trend toward microcephaly in alcohol-treated rats, in the absence of permanent effects on body weight in these animals, suggested that alcohol levels in rats that mimic moderate social drinking and binge drinking in the human do indeed produce a degree of microcephaly.

Body weights in alcohol-treated animals were reduced by only about one third as much as in malnutrition during the same time period (Culley & Lineberger, 1968). Brain weight reduction in the alcohol-treated animals was comparable to that observed by Culley and Lineberger in malnourished animals. By 70 days of age body weight in both alcohol-treated groups had caught up completely with that of controls. However, brain weight was decreased just as significantly at 70 days as it had been at 17 days of age. In malnourished animals, neither body nor brain weight caught up by 110 days of age (Culley & Lineberger, 1968).

Therefore the complete catch-up in body weight by 70 days of age in these animals suggested that the brain deficits were because of the pharmacological effects of alcohol rather than alcohol-induced malnutrition. Thus, alcohol exposure during the critically vulnerable brain growth spurt was reflected in altered whole brain and regional brain weights, regardless of how precisely nutritional status was controlled in alcohol-treated animals.

Although animal findings are not conclusive for the human, it is wise to consider the potential danger of alcohol exposure of the human brain during the brain growth spurt. Insofar as extrapolation is permissible, moderate social drinking or binge drinking by women during the third trimester of pregnancy or during lactation may disrupt normal synaptogenesis or normal blood–brain barrier development, which also occurs during the brain growth spurt. The effect of alcohol on blood–brain barrier development has not been reported. Disrupted or leaky blood–brain barrier tight junctions (the point at which capillary endothelial cells are sealed together), however, would affect synaptogenesis adversely.

Recently, Mills, Graubard, Harley, Rhoads, and Berendes (1984) reported on a prospective study of 31,604 pregnancies from 1974 through 1977. They observed that the percentage of newborns below the 10th percentile of weight for gestational age increased sharply with increasing maternal alcohol intake. Also, they found that consumption of one or two drinks daily was associated with a substantially increased risk of producing a growth-retarded infant. Because no safe level of alcohol intake has been established, Mills et al. (1984) advised that pregnant women limit alcoholic beverage intake to an occasional drink or at least not more than one drink per day. In view of their findings that one to two drinks a day were associated with significant risk, allowing one drink a day seems questionable. Their data did not permit assessment of either binge drinking or drinking beyond the first trimester of pregnancy. The fact that they looked only at the effects of drinking during the first trimester suggests that Mills et al. (1984) saw no need to evaluate the effects of alcohol exposure during the brain growth spurt. The animal data described above suggested a need for further studies of these effects.

Insofar as extrapolation is permitted, the disproportionate severity of the observed cerebellar effects in rats suggests implications for both the neuromotor and mental health of affected children. Berntson and Torello (1982) pointed out that ascending paleocerebellar limbic projections modulate mechanisms involved in motivation, emotional behaviors, and behavioral integration. Cerebellar damage, therefore, may be reflected not only in altered motor, sensory, and autonomic functions but also in disturbances of emotion, motivation, and behavior.

Synaptic alterations in brainstem respiratory centers may result from low blood alcohol concentrations during the brain growth spurt. Could these increase the risk of the sudden infant death syndrome (SIDS)? Although SIDS is the leading cause of death during the first postnatal year (Merritt & Valdes-Dapena, 1984), its etiology and neuropathology remain unknown. In the absence of infectious or chemical stress, subtle brainstem pathology might cause no apparent problem during infancy. If the stress of an acute upper respiratory infection were superimposed on an already compromised regulatory system, an infant's capacity to cope might be exceeded. Further, the depressant effects of alcohol in medications used to treat upper respiratory or other minor illnesses might suffice to tip the balance, allowing SIDS to occur.

ETHANOL AND LOW THYROXINE DURING ONTOGENY

Animal experiments have provided evidence that exposure of the brain during the brain growth spurt to low thyroxine levels, alone or in combination with alcohol or any central nervous system depressant, may increase the risk of SIDS. Brain changes that occurred in experimental animals from low thyroxine levels during the brain growth spurt include: (a) a decrease in mean cell size with an increase in cellular numerical density; (b) a hypoplastic axonal network; (c) a reduction in dendritic branching; (d) an abnormal distribution of dendritic spines; (e) decreased synaptic connectivity; and (f) altered vascularity (Eayrs, 1954, 1971; Eayrs & Goodhead, 1959).

These changes may be related to any of a diverse multiplicity of thyroxine effects on RNA and protein synthesis (Legrand, Clos, & Legrand, 1982). Hamburgh (1969) observed that low thyroxine during brain ontogeny resulted in decreased brain vascularization. If brainstem vascularity or synaptic and/or blood–brain barrier development are affected, then the risk of SIDS may be increased. Walsh (1986) observed that alcohol 0.6 g/kg body weight (used in the diluent for isopropylnorepinephrine) caused apnea frequently in hypothyroid rats but infrequently in control animals. Alcohol 0.6 g/kg in a rat is approximately equivalent to alcohol 0.2 g/kg in the human and is comparable to the amount of ethanol in an infant's dose of an elixir containing 18% alcohol.

Several studies on the effects of low maternal blood alcohol concentrations on fetal breathing were conducted on women (light social drinkers) at 37 to 40 weeks gestation. Real-time ultrasonic scanning was used prior to and after maternal ingestion of either 31 ml (one ounce) of vodka in diet ginger ale (Fox et al., 1978) or .25 g alcohol per kg body weight (1.5 ounces of vodka for a 125-lb woman) (Lewis & Boylan, 1979; McLeod et al., 1983, 1984). Within 30 minutes after the ingestion of alcohol, fetal respiratory movements in all subjects virtually were abolished and remained so throughout the

3 hours of monitoring. This result illustrates the extreme sensitivity of the brainstem respiratory center to alcohol during the third trimester. The resulting depression of feedback to the brainstem respiratory centers could interfere with synaptic maturation.

Clearly, relatively low intensity and/or short duration of alcohol exposure during critically vulnerable phases of brain ontogeny may result in subtle synaptic biochemical alterations. The dosages used in these human studies produced blood alcohol concentrations similar to those associated with moderate social drinking. Birth weight is significantly less in offspring of women who consume one to two drinks per day (Mills et al., 1984). Low birth weight has been associated with subtle behavioral and educational handicaps.

SUMMARY AND IMPLICATIONS
FOR NURSING RESEARCH

Synaptic integrity is essential for information processing and interneuronal communication in the central nervous system. Alcohol-induced synaptic disruption may be reflected in abnormal neurological function and altered mental and behavioral development. Perhaps the majority of people are somewhat brain-damaged given that the developing brain is so vulnerable to insult and so precisely, precariously programmed that few individuals are able to survive ontogeny unscathed by chemical or other stressors. Fortunately, the human brain is sufficiently complex that attainment of 90% of its potential is sufficient for most people to enjoy an acceptable quality of life. What might be the outcome of increasing the average human potential by 5%? To answer this question, new knowledge needs to be generated through research and applied to nursing work, particularly in the arena of child health and human development.

Further research is indicated in the area of maternal-child health concerning the use of alcoholic beverages or medications containing ethanol, as well as other central nervous system depressants, by pregnant and lactating women and the administration of these substances to children, particularly those under two years of age. Epidemiological studies are needed to determine whether or not there is a correlation between drinking patterns and/or use patterns of central nervous system depressants perinatally and the incidence of developmental behavioral disorders and SIDS. Additional studies are needed to determine whether or not an interaction of the effects of low blood alcohol concentrations and low thyroxine increases the risk of SIDS. Both animal and human studies are needed to answer the question as to whether exposure of the brain during the brain growth spurt affects synaptic systems (presynaptic and postsynaptic receptor numbers and/or binding capacity, neurotransmitter synthesis, storage, release, reuptake, and disposition) in a manner such as to alter responsiveness to alcohol and other drugs during juvenile and adult life.

REFERENCES

Alpert, J. J., Day, N., Dooling, E., Hingson, R., Oppenheimer, E., Rosett, H. L., Weiner, L., & Zukerman, B. (1981). Maternal alcohol consumption and newborn assessment: Methodology of the Boston City Hospital prospective study. *Neurobehavioral Toxicology and Teratology, 3,* 187–194.

Altman, J. (1969). Autoradiographic and histological studies of postnatal neurogenesis: III. Dating the time of production and onset of differentiation of cerebellar microneurons in rats. *Journal of Comparative Neurology, 136,* 269–294.

Altman, J. (1972a). Postnatal development of the cerebellar cortex in the rat: I. The external germinal layer and the transitional molecular layer. *Journal of Comparative Neurology, 145,* 353–398.

Altman, J. (1972b). Postnatal development of the cerebellar cortex in the rat: II. Phases in the maturation of Purkinje cells and of the molecular layer. *Journal of Comparative Neurology, 145,* 399–464.

Altman, J. (1972c). Postnatal development of the cerebellar cortex in the rat: III. Maturation of the components of the granular layer. *Journal of Comparative Neurology, 145,* 465–514.

American Academy of Pediatrics. (1984). Ethanol in liquid preparations intended for children. *Pediatrics, 73,* 405–407.

Andersson, K. (1982). Pharmacological inhibition of uterine activity. *Acta Obstetricia and Gynecologica Scandinavica, 108*(Suppl. 1), 17–23.

Barnes, D. E., & Walker, D. W. (1981). Prenatal ethanol exposure permanently reduces the number of pyramidal neurons in rat hippocampus. *Developmental Brain Research, 1,* 333–340.

Berntson, G. G., & Torello, M. W. (1982). Paleocerebellum in the integration of behavioral function. *Physiological Psychology, 10,* 2–12.

Burns, E. M., Kruckeberg, T. W., Kanak, M. F., & Stibler, H. (1986). Ethanol exposure during brain ontogeny: Some long-term effects. *Neurobehavioral Toxicology and Teratology, 8,* 383–389.

Burns, E. M., Kruckeberg, T. W., Stibler, H., Cerven, E., & Borg, S. (1984). Ethanol exposure during brain growth spurt. *Teratology, 29,* 251–258.

Burry, R. W., Kniss, D. A., & Scribner, L. R. (1984). Mechanisms of synapse formation and maturation. In D. G. Jones (Ed.), *Current topics in research on synapses* (Vol. 1) (pp. 1–51). New York: Alan R. Liss.

Caritis, S. N., Carson, D., Greebon, D., McCormick, M., Edelstone, D. I., & Mueller-Heuback, E. (1982). A comparison of terbutaline and ethanol in treatment of preterm labor. *American Journal of Obstetrics and Gynecology, 142,* 183–190.

Caritis, S. N., Edelstone, D. I., & Mueller-Heubach, E. (1979). Pharmacologic inhibition of preterm labor. *American Journal of Obstetrics and Gynecology, 133,* 557–578.

Clarren, S. K., Alvord, E. C., Sumi, S. M., Streissguth, A. P., & Smith, D. W. (1978). Brain malformations related to prenatal exposure to ethanol. *Journal of Pediatrics, 92,* 64–67.

Clarren, S. K., & Smith, D. W. (1978). The Fetal Alcohol Syndrome. *The New England Journal of Medicine, 298,* 1063–1067.

Cook, L. N., Shott, R. J., & Andrews, B. F. (1975). Acute transplacental ethanol intoxication. *American Journal of Diseases of Children, 129,* 1075–1076.

Culley, W. J., & Lineberger, R. O. (1968). Effect of undernutrition on the size and composition of the rat brain. *Journal of Nutrition, 96,* 375–381.

Department of Health and Human Services. (1987). *Sixth special report to the U.S. Congress on alcohol and health* (DHHS Publication No. 87-1519). Washington, DC: U.S. Government Printing Office.

Dobbing, J. (1971). Undernutrition and the developing brain. In R. Paoletti & A. N. Davison (Eds.), *Chemistry and brain development. Advances in experimental medicine and biology* (Vol. 13) (pp. 399–412). New York: Plenum Press.

Dobbing, J. (1974). The later growth of the brain and its vulnerability. *Pediatrics, 53,* 2–6.

Dobbing, J., & Sands, J. (1971). Undernutrition and the developing brain. In R. Paoletti & A. N. Davison (Eds.), *Chemistry and brain development. Advances in experimental medicine and biology* (Vol. 13) (pp. 399–412). New York: Plenum Press.

Dobbing, J., & Sands, J. (1979). Comparative aspects of the brain growth spurt. *Early Human Development, 3,* 79–83.

Dobbing, J., & Smart, J. L. (1973). Early undernutrition, brain development and behavior. In S. A. Barnett (Ed.), *Ethology and development. Clinics in developmental medicine* (Vol. 47) (pp. 16–36). Philadelphia: Lippincott.

Dow, K. E., & Riopelle, R. J. (1985). Ethanol neurotoxicity: Effects on neurite formation and neurotrophic factor production in vitro. *Science, 228,* 591–593.

Dreosti, I. E. (1984). Interactions between trace elements and alcohol in rats. In R. Porter, M. O'Connor, & J. Whelan (Eds.). *CIBA foundation symposium 105: Mechanisms of alcohol damage in utero* (pp. 103–123). London: The Pitman Press.

Eayrs, J. T. (1954). The vascularity of the cerebral cortex in normal and cretinous rats. *Journal of Anatomy, 88,* 164–173.

Eayrs, J. T. (1971). Thyroid and the developing brain: Anatomical and behavioral effects. In M. Hamburgh & E. J. W. Barrington (Eds.), *Hormones in development* (pp. 345–355). New York: Appleton-Century-Crofts.

Eayrs, J. T., & Goodhead, B. (1959). Postnatal development of the cerebral cortex in the rat. *Anatomy, 93*, 385–402.

Edelman, G. M. (1976). Surface modulation in cell recognition and cell growth. Some new hypotheses on phenotypic alteration and transmembranous control of cell surface receptors. *Science, 192*, 218–226.

Edelman, G. M. (1983). Cell adhesion molecules. *Science, 219*, 450–457.

Edelman, G. M. (1985). Cell adhesion and the molecular processes of morphogenesis. *Annual Review of Biochemistry, 54*, 135–169.

Ford, D. H., & Cramer, E. B. (1977). Developing nervous system in relation to thyroid hormones. In G. D. Grave (Ed.), *Thyroid hormones and brain development* (pp. 1–18). New York: Raven Press.

Fox, H. E., Steinbrecher, M., Pressel, D., Inglis, J., Medvid, L., & Angel, E. (1978). Maternal ethanol ingestion and the occurrence of human fetal breathing movements. *American Journal of Obstetrics and Gynecology, 132*, 354–358.

Fuchs, A. R., & Fuchs, F. (1981). Ethanol for prevention of preterm birth. *Seminars in Perinatology, 5*, 236–251.

Fuchs, F., Fuchs, A. R., Lauersen, N. H., & Zervoudakis, I. A. (1979). Treatment of pre-term labour with ethanol. *Danish Medical Bulletin, 26*, 123–124.

Hall, K., & Sara, V. R. (1983). Serum growth factors. *Vitamins and Hormones, 40*, 175–233.

Hamburgh, M. (1969). The role of thyroid and growth hormones in neurogenesis. *Current Topics in Developmental Biology, 4*, 109–148.

Hanson, J. W., Streissguth, A. P., & Smith, D. W. (1978). The effects of moderate alcohol consumption during pregnancy on fetal growth and morphogenesis. *Journal of Pediatrics, 92*, 457–460.

Hunt, W. A. (1985). *Alcohol and biological membranes.* New York: Guilford Press.

Inomata, K., Nasu, F., & Tanaka, H. (1987). Decreased density of synaptic formation in the frontal cortex of neonatal rats exposed to ethanol in utero. *International Journal of Developmental Neuroscience, 5*, 455–460.

Ito, M. (1984). Purkinje cells: Morphology and development. *The cerebellum and neural control* (pp. 21–39). New York: Raven Press.

Jones, K. L., & Smith, D. W. (1973). Recognition of the fetal alcohol syndrome in early infancy. *Lancet, 2*, 999–1001.

Jones, K. L., Smith, D. W., Streissguth, A. P., & Myrianthopoulos, N. C. (1974). Outcome in offspring of chronic alcoholic women. *Lancet, 1*, 2076–2078.

Kerfoot, K. M., Kruckeberg, T. W., & Burns, E. M. (1985). Maternal ethanol consumption and levels of ethanol in breast milk. *Proceedings of the 34th International Congress on Alcoholism and Drug Dependence* (p. 124). Calgary, Alberta, 1985.

Kesaniemi, Y. A. (1974). Ethanol and acetaldehyde in the milk and peripheral blood of lactating women after ethanol consumption. *Journal of Obstetrics and Gynecology, 81*, 84–86.

Kruckeberg, T. W., Gaetano, P. K., Burns, E. M., Stibler, H., Cerven, E., & Borg, S. (1984). Ethanol in preweanling rats with dams: Body temperature unaffected. *Neurobehavioral Toxicology and Teratology, 6*, 307–312.

Landesman-Dwyer, S. (1981). The relationship of children's behavior to maternal alcohol consumption. In A. L. Abel (Ed.), *Fetal alcohol syndrome* (Vol. II) (pp. 127–148). Boca Raton, FL: CRC Press.

Landesman-Dwyer, S., & Ragozin, A. S. (1981). Behavioral correlates of prenatal alcohol exposure: A four-year follow-up study. *Neurobehavioral Toxicology and Teratology, 3,* 187–194.

Legrand, C., Clos, J., & Legrand, J. (1982). Influence of altered thyroid and nutritional states on early histogenesis of rat cerebellar cortex with special reference to synaptogenesis. *Reproduction, Nutrition, and Development, 22,* 201–208.

Lemire, R. J., Loeser, J. D., Leech, R. W., & Alvord, E. C., Jr. (1975). *Normal and abnormal development of the human nervous system.* New York: Harper & Row.

Lewis, P. J., & Boylan, P. (1979). Alcohol and fetal breathing. *Lancet, 1,* 388.

Lyon, B. L., & Werner, J. S. (1987). Stress. In H. H. Werley & J. J. Fitzpatrick (Eds.), *Annual Review of Nursing Research* (Vol. 2) (pp. 3–22). New York: Springer Publishing.

Mason, S. T. (1981). Noradrenaline in the brain: Progress in theories of function. *Progress in Neurobiology, 16,* 263–303.

McLeod, W., Brien, J., Carmichael, L., Probert, C., Steenaart, N., & Patrick, J. (1984). Maternal glucose injections do not alter the suppression of fetal breathing following maternal ethanol ingestion. *American Journal of Obstetrics and Gynecology, 148,* 634–639.

McLeod, W., Brien, J., Loomis, C., Carmichael, L., Probert, C., & Patrick, J. (1983). Effect of maternal ethanol ingestion on fetal breathing movements, gross body movements, and heart rate at 37–40 weeks gestation. *American Journal of Obstetrics and Gynecology, 145,* 251–257.

Merritt, T. A., & Valdes-Dapena, M. (1984). Sudden infant death research update. *Pediatric Annals, 13,* 193–207.

Mills, J. L., Graubard, B. I., Harley, E. E., Rhoads, G. G., & Berendes, H. W. (1984). Maternal alcohol consumption and birth weight: How much drinking during pregnancy is safe? *Journal of the American Medical Association, 252,* 1875–1879.

Moore, K. L. (1977). *The developing human: Clinically oriented embryology* (2nd ed.) (pp. 33–95, 319–358). Philadelphia: Saunders.

Peden, V. H., Sammon, T. J., & Downey, D. A. (1973). Intravenously induced infantile intoxication with ethanol. *Fetal and Neonatal Medicine, 82,* 490–493.

Randall, C. L. (1977). Teratogenic effects of *in utero* ethanol exposure. In K. Blum (Ed.), *Alcohol and opiates* (pp. 91–108). New York: Academic Press.

Randall, C. L., Anton, R. F., & Becker, H. C. (1987). Alcohol, pregnancy, and prostaglandins. *Alcoholism: Clinical and Experimental Research, 11,* 32–36.

Randall, C. L., & Riley, E. P. (1984). Alcohol, pregnancy, babies: An up-date on the latest research—FAS/FAE. *Focus on Family and Chemical Dependency, 7,* 35–37.

Randall, C. L., & Taylor, W. J. (1979). Prenatal ethanol exposure in mice: Teratogenic effects. *Teratology, 19,* 305–372.

Rothbard, J. B., Brakenbury, R., Cunningham, B. A., & Edelman, G. M. (1982). Differences in the carbohydrate structures of neural cell-adhesion of molecules from adult and embryonic chicken brains. *The Journal of Biological Chemistry, 257,* 11064–11069.

Samson, H. H., & Grant, K. A. (1985). Fetal alcohol effects: Alcohol and the developing nervous system of the rat. In S. Parvez, Y. Burov, H. Parvez, & E. Burns (Eds.), *Alcohol, nutrition and the nervous system* (pp. 1–36). Utrecht, The Netherlands: VNU Science Press.

Sands, J., & Dobbing, J. (1981). Nutritional growth restriction and catch-up failure. In M. Monset-Couchard & A. Minkowski (Eds.), *Physiological and biochemical basis for perinatal medicine* (pp. 245–249). Basel: S. Karger.

Sara, V. R., Gennser, G., & Persson, P. H. (1982). Somatomedins during pregnancy and their relationship to fetal growth. *Journal of Developmental Physiology, 4,* 184–194.

Sara, V. R., Hall, K., Rodeck, C. H., & Wetterberg, L. (1981). Human embryonic somatomedin. *Proceedings of the National Academy of Science, 78,* 3175–3179.

Sara, V. R., & Tham, A. (1985). Hormonal regulation of brain growth and the possible effects of alcohol. In U. Rydberg, C. Alling, J. Engel, B. Pernow, L. A. Pellborn, & S. Rossner (Eds.), *Alcohol and the developing brain* (pp. 27–34). New York: Raven Press.

Seiger, A., & Granholm, A. C. (1981). Thyroxin dependency of the developing locus coeruleus. *Cell and Tissue Research, 220,* 1–15.

Shaywitz, B. A., Griffieth, G. G., & Warshaw, J. B. (1979). Hyperactivity and cognitive deficits in developing rat pups born to alcoholic mothers: An experimental model of EFAS. *Neurobehavioral Toxicology, 1,* 113–122.

Sisenwein, F. E., Tejani, N. A., Boxer, H. S., & DiGiuseppo, R. (1983). Effects of maternal ethanol infusion during pregnancy on the growth and development of children of four to seven years of age. *American Journal of Obstetrics and Gynecology, 147,* 52–56.

Souney, P. F., Kaul, A. F., & Osathanondh, R. (1983). Pharmacology of preterm labor. *Clinical Pharmacology, 2,* 29–44.

Stibler, H., Burns, E. M., Kruckeberg, T. W., Cerven, E., & Borg, S. (1985). Changes of synaptosomal surface carbohydrates after ethanol exposure during synaptogenesis. In H. Parvez, E. Burns, Y. Burov, & S. Parvez (Eds.), *Progress in alcohol research* (pp. 37–49). Utrecht, Holland: VNU Science Press.

Stibler, H., Burns, E., Kruckeberg, T. W., Gaetano, P., Cerven, E., Borg, S., & Tabakoff, B. (1983). Effect of ethanol on synaptosomal sialic acid metabolism in the developing rat brain. *Journal of the Neurological Sciences, 59,* 21–35.

Strahlendorf, H. K., & Strahlendorf, J. C. (1983). Ethanol suppression of locus coeruleus neurons: Relevancy to the fetal alcohol syndrome. *Neurobehavioral Toxicology and Teratology, 5,* 221–224.

Streissguth, A. P. (1986). Fetal alcohol syndrome: An overview and implications for patient management. In N. J. Estes & M. E. Heinemann (Eds.), *Alcoholism: Development, consequences, and interventions* (3rd ed.) (pp. 195–206). St. Louis: Mosby.

Streissguth, A. P., & LaDue, R. A. (1985). Psychological and behavioral effects in children prenatally exposed to alcohol. *Alcohol Health and World Research, 10,* 6–12.

Tabakoff, B., Noble, E. P., & Warren, K. R. (1979). Alcohol, nutrition, and the brain. In R. J. Wurtman & J. J. Wurtman (Eds.), *Nutrition and the brain* (Vol. 4) (pp. 159–213). New York: Raven Press.

Timiras, P. S., Vernadakis, A., & Sherwood, N. M. (1968). Development and plasticity of the nervous system. In N. S. Assali (Ed.), *Biology of gestation* (pp. 261–319). New York: Academic Press.

Van Dongen, P. A. M. (1981). The human locus coeruleus in neurology and psychiatry. *Progress in Neurobiology, 17*, 97–139.

Van Dyke, V. C., Mackay, L., & Ziaylek, E. N. (1982). Management of severe feeding dysfunction in children with fetal alcohol syndrome. *Clinical Pediatrics, 21*, 336–339.

Vernadakis, A., & Woodbury, D. M. (1969). The developing animal as a model. *Epilepsia, 10*, 163–178.

Walsh, R. (1986). [Apnea in hypothyroid rats exposed to ethanol]. Unpublished raw data.

Warren, K. R. (1977). *Critical review of the fetal alcohol syndrome.* Rockville, MD: National Institute of Alcohol Abuse and Alcoholism, The National Clearinghouse for Alcohol Information.

Weiner, N. (1980). Norepinephrine, epinephrine, and the sympathomimetic amines. In A. G. Gilman, L. S. Goodman, & A. Gilman (Eds.), *The pharmacological basis of therapeutics* (6th ed.) (pp. 138–175). New York: Macmillan.

Weiner, L., & Larson, G. (1987). Clinical prevention of fetal alcohol effects— A reality. *Alcohol Health and Research World, 11*, 60–63.

West, J. R. (1987). Fetal alcohol-induced brain damage and the problem of determining temporal vulnerability: A review. *Alcohol and Drug Research, 7*, 423–441.

West, J. R., & Hamre, K. M. (1985). Effects of alcohol exposure during different periods of development: Changes in hippocampal mossy fibers. *Developmental Brain Research, 17*, 280–284.

West, J. R., Hodges, C. A., & Black, A. C. (1981). Prenatal exposure to ethanol alters the organization of hippocampal mossy fibers in rats. *Science, 211*, 957–959.

Wiener, S. G., Shoemaker, W. J., Koda, L. Y., & Bloom, F. E. (1981). Interaction of ethanol and nutrition during gestation: Influence on maternal and offspring development in the rat. *Journal of Pharmacology and Experimental Therapeutics, 216*, 572–579.

Chapter 4

Smoking Cessation:
Research on Relapse Crises

KATHLEEN A. O'CONNELL
MIDWEST RESEARCH INSTITUTE
AND SCHOOL OF NURSING
UNIVERSITY OF KANSAS MEDICAL CENTER

CONTENTS

The purpose of this chapter is to review that portion of the research on smoking cessation that deals with relapse crises. Nursing research on smoking has focused on the smoking behavior of nurses. Most of the studies of relapse crises have been conducted by nonnurses, and none of them have been published in nursing journals. However, the methodologies and the findings of the research on relapse crises have implications for research on health promotion and disease prevention, areas that have been recognized as major priorities in nursing research.

To place this review in context, a brief introduction to the findings in the general literature on smoking cessation is presented, and the nursing literature on smoking is discussed briefly. Thereafter the methods and findings of the research on relapse crises in smoking are presented. Major issues related to the research are discussed and implications for nursing research are addressed.

RESEARCH ON SMOKING CESSATION

Cigarette smoking has been cited as one of the major preventable causes of mortality and morbidity in the United States (U.S. Department of Health and Human Services [U.S. DHHS], 1982). Thus smoking behavior has been the focus of numerous health promotion efforts. Nurses, psychologists, physicians, and other health professionals have contributed to the large body of basic and applied studies on smoking behavior and smoking cessation. The cessation studies have shown that relapse is the most prevalent outcome of cessation attempts. Approximately 70% of the subjects relapse within 3 months of initiating a cessation attempt, and an additional 10 to 15% relapse between 3 and 12 months after initiation (Hunt, Barnett, & Branch, 1971; Marlatt & Gordon, 1985; Schwartz, 1969, 1987). Investigators have been unable to devise interventions that improve success rates above 40% at 1 year follow-up, and they have been largely unsuccessful in identifying smoker characteristics that are clinically useful in predicting success or failure in a cessation attempt. Although multivariate approaches often achieve statistically significant results, the amount of variance accounted for typically is low (i.e., less than 20%) (O'Connell, 1985; Swan et al., 1988; Swan, Parker, Carmelli, Rosenman, & Denk, 1985), and the results are inconsistent from study to study.

Because neither the intervention technique nor the personality of the smoker has been particularly useful in predicting successful long-term cessation, Marlatt and his colleagues turned their attention to the study of the relapse phenomenon (Cummings, Gordon, & Marlatt, 1980; Marlatt & Gordon, 1980). The descriptive and theoretical work of these investigators launched a group of studies that were focused on the relapse crises of individuals who were attempting to quit smoking. The results of those studies provided important clues about the process of smoking cessation (Curry et al., 1987; O'Connell & Martin, 1987).

NURSING RESEARCH ON SMOKING

Information for this section was gathered from a review of the nursing journal entries under *smoking* that were in the *Cumulative Index to Nursing and Allied Health Literature* for the years 1981 through 1987 and from the computerized search of nursing literature called *Nurse-Search*, using the term *smoking* for the years 1985 through the first half of 1988. This search revealed 23 studies published in nursing journals. Investigators in 18 (78%) of those studies were concerned with the smoking behavior of nurses. Only five of the studies were focused on nonnurse samples.

Most of the nursing research on the smoking behavior of nurses consisted of surveys about the prevalence of smoking among nurses and the percentages of nurses who were ex-smokers and relapsers (e.g., Feldman & Richard, 1986; Wagner, 1985). The focus on the smoking behavior of nurses was understandable, because a 1975 survey indicated that nurses had the highest rate of smoking among health care professionals (39%) (U.S. National Clearing House for Smoking and Health, 1976). This rate exceeded that of females in the general population by 10 percentage points. Thus there was considerable interest in the rates of smoking among nurses and the possible factors contributing to those rates, an interest that was also evident in nonnursing publications (e.g., Garfinkel & Stellman, 1986). However, these studies were mostly epidemiological in nature and made little contribution to an understanding of smoking behavior in general.

Studies published in nursing journals that were focused on nonnurse samples were likewise mostly descriptive of the prevalence of smoking behavior among various clinical samples (e.g., Black, 1984) with little attention to smoking cessation. An exception to this is the work of Wewers and Lenz (1987), who tested the power of a theoretical model to predict successful smoking cessation with 150 persons who had attended a smoking cessation clinic. None of the studies concerned relapse crises.

It should be noted, however, that studies by nurse investigators often appear in nonnursing publications and, therefore, are not included in this brief review of the nursing research on smoking. Such studies include work by Becker (Becker et al., 1986) and Wewers (1988) as well as my own work (O'Connell & Martin, 1987; O'Connell & Shiffman, 1988).

RELAPSE CRISES

Definitions

In order to define the term *relapse crisis*, it is necessary to define the terms *abstinence, temptation, lapse,* and *relapse.* Although some investigators have used reduction in smoking rate as the major outcome variable, most experts now agree that abstinence is the goal of smoking control programs (Ossip-Klein et al., 1986). *Abstinence* is defined as the state in which an individual refrains from *smoking* tobacco products for a period of at least 24 hours. Subjects who use smokeless tobacco (relatively rare among ex-smokers) and subjects who use nicotine gum (currently being used by an increasing number of individuals who are trying to quit smoking) usually are considered abstinent. For purposes of this review, a *temptation* (sometimes called a close call) is defined as a specific episode occurring after a period of voluntary abstinence during which an ex-smoker is tempted highly to smoke, but resists. A *lapse* (sometimes called a slip) is defined as an isolated smoking episode occurring after a period of voluntary abstinence that is not followed by continuous smoking. *Relapse* is defined as a smoking episode after a period of voluntary abstinence that is followed by a return to continuous smoking. A relapse crisis can be a temptation, lapse, or relapse. It should be noted that the term *crisis* is meant to convey the heightened vulnerability to relapse rather than periods of high stress. A significant proportion of relapse crises occur in situations characterized by low stress and positive mood.

Approach to the Review

This review included all reports of studies of relapse crises that appeared in a *PsychLit* computer search of *Psychological Abstracts* using the terms *smoking* and *relapse* from 1974 to June, 1988. In addition, the search was supplemented by the author's collection of published and unpublished papers that included investigations of relapse crises. It should be noted that not all studies that appeared under the terms smoking and relapse concerned actual relapse crises. Studies in which relapse to smoking was discussed without presentation of data on the actual relapse crises of the subjects were excluded from the review.

This chapter is organized using a topical approach that emphasizes the types of studies that have been done. The review begins with an overview of the methodologies used in these studies, after which three major topic areas are discussed: (a) classification of relapse crises, (b) responses to relapse crises, and (c) correlates of relapse crises. Finally, the strengths and weaknesses of the studies are examined.

Methods for Studying Relapse Crises

Investigations of relapse crises have been implemented with a standard methodology consisting of interviews conducted during or at varying periods of time after the relapse crises. The interviews typically included questions on the circumstances, environmental characteristics, and emotional states before and during the relapse crises. Many researchers also incorporated questions about the subjects' responses to the crises. Such responses including coping strategies, attributions for the causes of the crises, and affective reactions to the crises (as distinct from affects that precipitated the crises). Although some investigations were limited to subjects who had relapsed (e.g., Baer & Lichtenstein, 1988; Colletti, Supnick, & Rizzo, 1981; Cummings et al., 1980; Marlatt & Gordon, 1980; Sjoberg & Johnson, 1978), others included subjects reporting lapses and highly tempting situations in which smoking was resisted as well as subjects who relapsed (Curry & Marlatt, 1985; O'Connell & Martin, 1987; Shiffman, 1982). The final outcome of the smoking cessation attempt was also available for most studies.

Most of the methodologies were retrospective, with the subjects reporting on episodes that occurred several days to several months prior to the interviews. The major exceptions to this retrospective approach were several reports published by Shiffman (1982, 1984) on subjects who called a relapse prevention hotline and an investigation that required subjects to mail in a questionnaire immediately after a slip (Curry, Marlatt, & Gordon, 1987). The data-analytic approaches of the studies varied from simple descriptive techniques to log-linear and cluster analyses. Also, it should be noted that several of the reports included more than one type of study. For instance, a particular investigation may have included both a classification of relapse episodes and an analysis of responses to relapse episodes.

Classification of Relapse Crises

Two approaches to the classification of relapse episodes have been used. The most prevalent is an empirical approach that involves sorting the episodes on the basis of a scheme that is derived from the data itself. A theoretical approach that involves sorting the episodes according to predetermined theoretical constructs has been used less often.

Empirical Approaches.   Marlatt and his colleagues used a content analysis technique to devise a classification scheme to categorize relapse episodes in a variety of addictions (Cummings et al., 1980; Marlatt & Gordon, 1980). In their most extensive study (Cummings et al., 1980), 311 initial relapse episodes in drinking, smoking, compulsive gambling, excessive eating, and heroin addiction were classified. Although there was some variation, the pattern of results was surprisingly consistent across the different types of addictions. Of the 64 smokers in the study, 52% relapsed when they were experiencing negative emotional states, and 32% relapsed in response to direct or indirect social pressure to smoke. Colletti et al. (1981) found similar results with subjects who relapsed to smoking.

In a subsequent study O'Connell and Martin (1987) used the categorization scheme developed by Marlatt and his colleagues (Cummings, Marlatt, & Gordon, 1980) to compare three groups of subjects: (a) abstainers describing temptations ($n = 85$), (b) lapsers ($n = 60$), and (c) relapsers ($n = 451$). Analyses revealed that relapsers described significantly more situations characterized by withdrawal symptoms and other negative affect states than did lapsers or abstainers. Also, relapsers were significantly less likely to describe situations involving cigarette cues than were temporary lapsers and abstainers. Temporary lapsers and abstainers did not differ in the types of episodes they reported. These findings suggested that relapse episodes were qualitatively different from episodes in which subjects resisted smoking altogether or had a temporary lapse.

Using multiple variables, Shiffman (1982) classified the relapse crises of 183 subjects who called a relapse prevention hotline. He found that relapse crises were about equally likely to occur at any time during the waking day, the majority of the crises took place in subjects' homes, and other smokers were present in about one third of the cases. Eating (29% of the cases) was the most frequent activity that preceded the relapse crises, and about 20% of the crises involved the consumption of alcohol. Most of the relapse crises (71%) occurred in the presence of negative affect (dysphoric moods), and about half were associated with withdrawal symptoms. In 55% of the cases, the precipitating stimuli were identified as negative affect or severe stress. When Shiffman compared subjects who lapsed during the crises (40%) with those who resisted the temptation to smoke (60%), he found that the subjects did not differ on antecedent activities, affect, or amount of stress. Surprisingly, subjects who were experiencing withdrawal symptoms were significantly less likely to lapse than those without symptoms. Those in the presence of other smokers were significantly more likely to lapse than those who had not been with smokers. Lapses were significantly more likely to occur when alcohol was being consumed and when subjects were in bars and restaurants rather than at home or at work. Overall, however, Shiffman found that situational characteristics were less important than the subjects' coping responses in determining whether or not they smoked in the situations.

In a subsequent report, Shiffman (1986) used a cluster-analytic approach to combine the classification variables used in his 1982 study. This analysis yielded four clusters of situations: (a) upset (negative affect, usually at home, often alone), (b) work (tension at work settings with co-workers present), (c) social (with smokers, alcohol present, usually in a bar, restaurant, or friend's home); and (d) relaxation (at home, often after a meal with positive affect and others present). These clusters differed from each other on precessation motivations for smoking, indicating that subjects tended to have relapse crises in situations in which they had regularly smoked. Coping strategies also varied across the clusters.

Baer and Lichtenstein (1988) attempted to replicate Shiffman's cluster-analytic findings in their study of 176 subjects who relapsed after they had participated in smoking cessation programs. As a group, the subjects were similar to those in Shiffman's sample who had smoked during the relapse crises. However, the cluster-analytic solution did not resemble Shiffman's four-cluster solution. In addition, a split-half reliability procedure demonstrated that no reliable clusters could be identified in this data set. The findings of the study did suggest that stress, socializing with other smokers, and the consumption of food and alcohol often were associated with relapse.

Theoretical Approaches.   Only two groups of investigators have used a theoretical approach to classifying smoking relapse episodes. Sjoberg and Johnson (1978) presented a theoretical analysis of volitional breakdowns. In support of their theoretical formulations, the investigators presented a descriptive study of 10 subjects who relapsed to smoking. Nine of the subjects exhibited twisted reasoning as described in the theory, but the evidence was anecdotal, with no attention given to reliability of coding or to operational definitions of mood pressure or twisted thinking. Gerkovich, Potocky, O'Connell, and Cook (1989) used concepts from the theory of psychological reversals (Apter, 1982) to classify the relapse crises of 55 subjects who had attended smoking cessation programs. All subjects were interviewed 3 months after cessation. The sample was drawn from a larger study of relapse crises (O'Connell & Martin, 1987), so that about half (27) of the subjects had resisted the temptation to smoke and half (28) of the subjects had lapsed during the crises. It was hypothesized that highly tempting situations that took place in paratelic (sensation-oriented) states were more likely to result in lapses than those that took place in telic (goal-oriented) states. It was hypothesized further that highly tempting situations that occurred when the subject was in a negativistic state were more likely to result in lapses than when a subject was in a conformist state. Intercoder reliability was .96 for telic/paratelic states and .89 for negativistic/conformist states. Log-linear analyses revealed that the hypotheses were supported. In addition, when the telic/paratelic and negativistic/conformist dimensions were used together to classify the subjects according to whether they lapsed or abstained during the episodes, correct classifications were achieved for 93% of the episodes.

Responses to Relapse Crises

The second type of research on relapse crises deals with subjects' responses to those crises. Two types of responses are discussed: reactions to lapses and coping strategies used during relapse crises.

Reactions to Lapses.   Researchers in several studies have demonstrated that relapse rates for subjects who lapse were near 90% (Brandon, Tiffany, & Baker, 1986; O'Connell & Martin, 1987). In order to explain this phenomenon of a single lapse inexorably escalating into a full-blown relapse even after weeks or months of abstinence, Marlatt and his colleagues (Marlatt, 1985a; Marlatt & Gordon, 1980) posited that initial use of a substance after a period of voluntary abstinence likely would precipitate the "abstinence violation effect."

The abstinence violation effect is a combination of cognitive dissonance, causal attribution, and an affective reaction to the attribution. The ex-smoker who smokes a cigarette experiences dissonance. He is a nonsmoker and yet he is smoking. At the same time he is motivated to make an internal or personal attribution about the cause of the lapse. This causal attribution is likely to be characterized as stable ("It will always be this way"), global ("It will affect everything I do"), and uncontrollable. Thus the person who lapses would be likely to say, "I smoked because I never have been the kind of person who could quit a habit like smoking." Schoeneman and his colleagues (Schoeneman, Hollis, Stevens, Fischer, & Cheek, 1988) have termed this type of attribution *characterological self-blame*, a term used by Janoff-Bulman (1979) in a study of rape victims. Emotional reactions to this type of attribution often involve self-blame and guilt, which serve to reduce self-efficacy and future striving for a goal. The combination of the motivation to reduce the dissonance and the decreased self-efficacy work together to cause the ex-smoker to resume his or her previous habit. Several investigators have supported this formulation (Curry et al., 1987; O'Connell & Martin, 1987; Schoeneman et al., 1988). However, the abstinence violation effect has not been supported in at least one study (Brandon et al., 1986).

Coping Strategies.   The abstinence violation effect is part of a cognitive-behavioral model of relapse that Marlatt and his associates have developed (Marlatt, 1985b; Marlatt & Gordon, 1980). The model illustrates a series of events that are posited to ensue when the individual encounters a high-risk situation. If the individual engages in a coping response, increased self-efficacy (Bandura, 1977) will be experienced, and this will lead to decreased probability of relapse. If the individual does not engage in a coping response, decreased self-efficacy will be experienced. In addition, the individual may remember selectively and focus on the positive effects of the target substance. If these effects are seen as helpful in increasing one's ability to cope with the stressful situation, and the individual's self-efficacy for dealing with the situation without the substance is undermined sufficiently, then initial use of the substance will ensue. The initial use of the substance will lead to the abstinence violation effect, which will predispose the subject to a full-blown relapse.

Although evidence supporting the entire cognitive-behavioral model of smoking relapse has not been presented, findings from several studies have supported parts of the model. Evidence for the abstinence violation effect has been presented previously. In addition, the importance of coping responses has been addressed in several studies. Shiffman (1984) studied the coping responses during relapse crises of subjects who called his hotline. Findings of his previous study (Shiffman, 1982) were cross-validated on a new sample of 75 subjects. His findings showed that any type of coping response was more effective than no coping response in helping to resist the temptation to smoke. Although the number of coping responses was not related to outcome of the relapse crises, the type of coping response did influence outcomes. Subjects who used a combination of cognitive and behavioral responses were more likely to resist smoking than subjects who used only one type of strategy. A subsequent analysis of the same data set (Shiffman & Jarvik, 1987) revealed that coping responses were more likely to be performed in the early phases of abstinence and in situations in which subjects had smoked habitually.

Shiffman's studies of individuals who called a hotline in response to relapse crises have been criticized because the subjects were engaging in a coping strategy by calling the hotline and therefore might have different coping behaviors than other types of subjects. However, in a study of unaided quitters (i.e., individuals who did not go through a formalized smoking cessation program), Curry and Marlatt (1985) replicated some of Shiffman's findings. Compared to relapsers, those who resisted smoking were significantly more likely to report the use of coping strategies during the relapse crises.

Correlates of Relapse Crises

The third type of research on relapse crises concerns variables that are related to experiencing certain types of crises. If individuals who are particularly vulnerable to having certain types of relapse crises could be identified, then special interventions might be developed.

Several investigators have addressed this issue by studying the similarities between different relapse crises experienced by the same subject. Conflicting results have been obtained. For instance, Shiffman (in press) found little evidence for trans-situational consistency in his study of successive relapse crises of 57 hotline callers. In their study of the relapse episodes of 176 subjects, Baer and Lichtenstein (1988) found that prior relapse episodes following a previous cessation attempt were not similar to current relapse episodes. However, lapse episodes that occurred during the current cessation attempt were related highly to current relapse episodes. Differences in these findings may have reflected the different study samples (hotline callers versus participants in smoking cessation programs) and different cessation outcomes (mixed abstainers, lapsers, and relapsers versus relapsers only).

Another approach has been to determine if certain subject characteristics predisposed ex-smokers to experience certain types of relapse crises. O'Connell and Shiffman (1988) showed that individuals who had smoked in negative affect situations prior to their quit attempt, as measured by the Motivations for Smoking Scale (Ikard, Green, & Horn, 1969), were significantly more likely to experience relapse crises in negative affect states than were subjects who had not smoked in negative affect states. Shiffman (1986) found similar relationships between prior smoking behavior and the four clusters he identified. However, Baer and Lichtenstein (1988) found no relationship between negative affect smoking and type of relapse crises. Moreover, relapse crises also were unrelated to prior measures of self-efficacy, perceived stress, and nicotine addiction.

STRENGTHS, WEAKNESSES, AND ISSUES

The literature on relapse crises has improved understanding of the relapse process and of precipitants of relapse. Some of the findings have been used in the design of intervention studies (Brown, Lichtenstein, McIntyre, & Harrington-Kostur, 1984; Cooney & Kopel, 1980; Cooney, Kopel, & McKeon, 1982; Hall, Rugg, Tunstall, & Jones, 1984; Supnick & Colletti, 1984). Yet none of the intervention studies included specific investigations of relapse crises. Thus the effects of specific interventions on ex-smokers' responses to relapse crises needs to be explored further.

One of the major limitations of the studies on relapse crises involves the types of samples that have been studied. Many of the studies of relapse crises have been focused only on those subjects who smoked during the crises. Without a comparison group of subjects who resisted the temptation to smoke, the findings on the types of situations that predispose subjects to engage in the initial smoking episode are difficult to interpret.

When studies that are limited to initial smoking episodes are designed to compare lapse with relapse episodes, valuable information can be produced. The major problem with these studies, however, is that the lapses without subsequent relapses are relatively rare (about 10% of all subjects who experience an initial smoking episode). Therefore, studies with large initial sample sizes frequently yield small numbers of lapsers, thus limiting the power of statistical analyses.

Although the addition of temptations (crises that did not lead to smoking) to the research on relapse crises would have improved understanding of the factors that led to initial smoking, this procedure has some methodological problems as well. O'Connell and Martin (1987) showed that temptation situations described by the subjects were significantly more recent than were lapse situations. Apparently subjects tended to forget remote situations in which they overcame the urge to smoke and tended to report situations that occurred in the recent past. Thus memory factors may operate differentially in lapse and temptation situations.

Other methodological issues are also important in research of this type. First, the self-report nature of the research has implications for the validity of the findings. Objective indices to verify abstinence (e.g., salivary cotinine, expired air carbon monoxide, corroborative reports from subjects' acquaintances) have become standard in smoking research. Such indices have been used in some of the studies of relapse crises that included abstainers. However, the reports that included ex-smokers calling a relapse prevention hotline included neither objective reports of abstinence nor measures of final outcome of the cessation attempt.

Self-report also may affect the data concerning the relapse crises themselves. Subjects may be reluctant to tell investigators their true feelings or actual behavior during the crises. They may inflate their reports of using coping strategies in order to make it appear that they really did try to resist the temptation. Memory factors may play an important role in what is reported. In addition, subjects may tend to re-evaluate certain aspects of relapse crises in light of their current behavior. For instance, attributions may not be the cause of the relapse, but rather the effect of observing that one has returned to regular smoking.

It should be noted also that several of the research reports on relapse crises are based on the same data sets. For instance, in the research on relapse crises reported by Shiffman (Shiffman, 1982, 1984, 1986, in press; Shiffman & Jarvik, 1987) the same sample or extensions of the same sample were used. The three studies reported by O'Connell were performed using the same sample of subjects (Gerkovich et al., 1989; O'Connell & Martin, 1987; O'Connell & Shiffman, 1988). Thus eight of the reported studies are based on only two separate data sets. Therefore, the findings presented here may be affected particularly by specific sample characteristics. Clearly, additional research on different samples is needed.

Despite these limitations, the research on relapse crises has led to a deeper understanding of the phenomenon of behavior change. Findings have indicated that such change is not only a function of personality and treatment characteristics but also a function of how individuals respond to specific high-risk situations.

IMPLICATIONS FOR NURSING RESEARCH

Nursing research on smoking cessation has been sparse. However, with the increasing emphasis in nursing on health promotion and disease prevention, more nursing investigations on smoking are warranted. Specifically, nursing research on smoking should focus on the smoking behavior of subjects other than nurses. In addition, more work is needed on the factors influencing successful cessation among clinical populations and on low-income and minority groups. Given the frequent contact of both primary care and community health nurses with such populations, it would appear that nurse investigators have a unique opportunity to contribute to the literature in these areas.

Schwartz (1987) has noted that the role of nurses in helping patients quit smoking has not been studied adequately. The types of smoking cessation interventions that could be studied by nurse investigators are varied (see Schwartz, 1987, for a comprehensive review of the types of interventions). Nursing intervention techniques that are based on current behavioral and pharmacological (i.e., nicotine replacement therapies) approaches could be useful. Minimal interventions delivered in physicians' offices might be adapted for delivery by nurses in outpatient settings. Innovative techniques that meet the needs of specific populations (e.g., pregnant smokers, diabetic smokers) would also be warranted. The results of the research on relapse underscore the challenge that such intervention programs present. Relapse is prevalent, underreporting of smoking is common, and short-term interventions that do not provide follow-up almost certainly are doomed to failure. Intervention techniques aimed at hospitalized patients, who are usually acutely ill, present special challenges. Such patients may be highly motivated to quit smoking during their hospitalization. However, their physical conditions usually preclude the type of intensive training that many intervention programs use. Shortened hospital stays further reduce the opportunity to administer hospital-based interventions.

Additional research on relapse crises similar to the studies reviewed in this chapter are needed. The relationships between temptations to smoke and fluctuations in disease states have yet to be investigated. For instance, do patients with pulmonary disease experience increased urges to smoke when their symptoms increase or when they abate? Other needed research includes investigations that elucidate the types of strategies that are used for overcoming the urge to smoke and the types of situations where such coping strategies are likely to be employed or ignored.

In order for nursing research on smoking to build on the available evidence, certain methodological considerations are important. First, adequate sample sizes are necessary. Attrition is high in smoking cessation programs. Differences between treatment approaches are likely to be small. Thus large samples are usually necessary. Second, objective indices of smoking cessation are necessary elements of an adequate appraisal of smoking cessation interventions (Ossip-Klein et al., 1986). Objective indices include biochemical measures and collateral reports. The choice of an objective index depends on the purposes of the study, but attention must be given to the sensitivity and specificity of the method chosen. Third, adequate long-term follow-up is necessary to assess the effects of any intervention program. Relapse rates often rise quickly after the intensive portions of the programs are completed. Thus, end-of-treatment success rates are inadequate measures of outcome. Most experts recommend follow-up periods of 6 to 12 months.

In addition to its implications for smoking, research on relapse crises also has implications for research in other areas of health behavior. Recent investigations have shown that success in changing health behavior often comes after a number of relapses and that there are commonalities across different types of behavior change (Brownell, Marlatt, Lichtenstein, & Wilson, 1986; Schachter, 1982). Thus some of the findings in the smoking research are applicable to research in other areas. For instance, Grilo, Shiffman, and Wing (1989) have studied the relapse crises experienced by persons with diabetes who are on weight-reduction diets. Although studying dieting requires some changes in methodology (e.g., the definition of a relapse is necessarily different, since abstinence cannot be a goal), the findings of the study are generally consistent with some of the findings on smoking relapse crises. Applications of the methodology to research on other health behaviors like exercise and taking medication are also possible.

Research on relapse crises has grown out of the realization that long-term behavior change is a complex phenomenon. Simple studies on treatments, traits, and outcomes cannot account for meaningful proportions of variance. More emphasis must be given to the process of behavior change as well as to the maintenance of change. Research on situations in which patients are tempted to abandon newly acquired behaviors may be especially useful in elucidating specific problems that must be overcome in maintaining the changes in lifestyle. With their knowledge of clinical issues and their access to clinical populations, nurse investigators who are moving into health promotion areas have a unique opportunity. If they acknowledge the complexity of behavior change while applying their own theories and models, nurses can improve health promotion outcomes for their clients, and they also can make a substantial contribution to the understanding of behavior change.

REFERENCES

Apter, M. J. (1982). *The experience of motivation: The theory of psychological reversals.* London: Academic Press.

Baer, J. S., & Lichtenstein, E. (1988). Classification and prediction of smoking relapse episodes: An exploration of individual differences. *Journal of Consulting and Clinical Psychology, 56,* 104–110.

Bandura, A. (1977). Self-efficacy: Toward a unifying theory of behavioral change. *Psychological Review, 84,* 191–215.

Becker, D. M., Myers, A. H., Sacci, M., Weida, S., Swank, R., Levine, D. M., & Pearson, T. A. (1986). Smoking behavior and attitudes toward smoking among hospital nurses. *American Journal of Public Health, 76,* 1449–1451.

Black, P. (1984). Towards tomorrow's world: Who stops smoking in pregnancy? *Nursing Times, 80*(19), 59–61.

Brandon, T. H., Tiffany, S. T., & Baker, T. B. (1986). The process of smoking relapse. In F. M. Tims & C. G. Leukefeld (Eds.), *Relapse and recovery in drug abuse* (NIDA Research Monograph No. 72) (pp. 104–117). Rockville, MD: United States Public Health Service.

Brown, R. A., Lichtenstein, E., McIntyre, K. O., & Harrington-Kostur, J. (1984). Effects of nicotine fading and relapse prevention on smoking cessation. *Journal of Consulting and Clinical Psychology, 52,* 307–308.

Brownell, K. D., Marlatt, G. A., Lichtenstein, E., & Wilson, G. T. (1986). Understanding and preventing relapse. *American Psychologist, 41,* 765–782.

Colletti, G., Supnick, J. A., & Rizzo, A. A. (1981, August). *An analysis of relapse determinants.* Paper presented at the meeting of the American Psychological Association, Los Angeles, CA.

Cooney, N. L., & Kopel, S. A. (1980, August). *Controlled relapse: A social learning approach to preventing smoking recidivism.* Paper presented at the meeting of the American Psychological Association, Montreal.

Cooney, N. L., Kopel, S. A., & McKeon, P. (1982, August). *Controlled relapse training and self-efficacy in smokers.* Paper presented at the meeting of the American Psychological Association, Washington, D.C.

Cummings, C., Gordon, J. R., & Marlatt, G. A. (1980). Relapse: Prevention and prediction. In W. R. Miller (Ed.), *The addictive disorders: Treatment of alcoholism, drug abuse, smoking, and obesity* (pp. 291–322). New York: Pergamon.

Curry, S., Marlatt, G. A., & Gordon, J. R. (1987). Abstinence violation effect: Validation of an attributional construct with smoking cessation. *Journal of Consulting and Clinical Psychology, 55,* 145–149.

Curry, S. G., & Marlatt, G. A. (1985). Unaided quitters' strategies for coping with temptations to smoke. In S. Shiffman & T. A. Wills (Eds.), *Coping and substance abuse* (pp. 243–265). Orlando, FL: Academic Press.

Feldman, B. M., & Richard, E. (1986). Prevalence of nurse smokers and variables identified with successful and unsuccessful smoking cessation. *Research in Nursing & Health, 9,* 131–138.

Garfinkel, L., & Stellman, S. D. (1986). Cigarette smoking among physicians, dentists, and nurses. *CA, 36*(1), 2–8.

Gerkovich, M. M., Potocky, M., O'Connell, K. A., & Cook, M. R. (1989). *Using the somatic modes of reversal theory to classify relapse crises of ex-smokers.* Paper presented at the Fourth International Conference on the Theory of Psychological Reversals, Athabasca, Alberta, Canada.

Grilo, S., Shiffman, S., & Wing, R. R. (1989). Relapse crises and coping among dieters. *Journal of Consulting and Clinical Psychology, 57*, 488–495.

Hall, S. M., Rugg, D., Tunstall, C., & Jones, R. T. (1984). Preventing relapse to cigarette smoking by behavioral skill training. *Journal of Consulting and Clinical Psychology, 52*, 372–382.

Hunt, W. A., Barnett, L. W., & Branch, L. G. (1971). Relapse rates in addiction programs. *Journal of Clinical Psychology, 27*, 455–456.

Ikard, F. F., Green, D., & Horn, D. (1969). A scale to differentiate between types of smoking as related to the management of affect. *International Journal of the Addictions, 4*, 649–659.

Janoff-Bulman, R. (1979). Characterological versus behavioral self blame: Inquiries into depression and rape. *Journal of Personality and Social Psychology, 37*, 1798–1809.

Marlatt, G. A. (1985a). Cognitive factors in the relapse process. In G. A. Marlatt & J. R. Gordon (Eds.), *Relapse prevention* (pp. 128–200). New York: Guilford.

Marlatt, G. A. (1985b). Relapse prevention: Theoretical rationale and overview of the model. In G. A. Marlatt & J. R. Gordon (Eds.), *Relapse prevention* (pp. 3–70). New York: Guilford.

Marlatt, G. A., & Gordon, J. R. (1980). Determinants of relapse: Implications for the maintenance of behavior change. In P. O. Davidson & S. M. Davidson (Eds.), *Behavioral medicine: Changing health lifestyles* (pp. 410–452). Elmsford, NY: Pergamon.

Marlatt, G. A., & Gordon, J. R. (Eds.). (1985). *Relapse prevention: Maintenance strategies in addictive behavior change.* New York: Guilford.

O'Connell, K. A. (1985, August). *Predictors of short-term and long-term smoking cessation.* Paper presented at the meeting of the American Psychological Association, Los Angeles, CA.

O'Connell, K. A., & Martin, E. J. (1987). Highly tempting situations associated with abstinence, temporary lapse, and relapse among participants in smoking cessation programs. *Journal of Consulting and Clinical Psychology, 55*, 367–371.

O'Connell, K. A., & Shiffman, S. (1988). Negative affect smoking and smoking relapse. *Journal of Substance Abuse, 1*, 25–33.

Ossip-Klein, D. J., Bigelow, G., Parker, S. R., Curry, S., Hall, S., & Kirkland, S. (1986). Classification and assessment of smoking behavior. *Health Psychology, 5*(Suppl.), 3–11.

Schachter, S. (1982). Recidivism and self-cure of smoking and obesity. *American Psychologist, 37*, 436–444.

Schoeneman, T. J., Hollis, J. F., Stevens, V. J., Fischer, K., & Cheek, P. R. (1988). Recovering stride versus letting it slide: Attributions for "slips" following smoking cessation treatment. *Psychology and Health, 2*, 335–347.

Schwartz, J. L. (1969). A critical review and evaluation of smoking control methods. *Public Health Reports, 84*, 483–506.

Schwartz, J. L. (1987). *Review and evaluation of smoking cessation methods: The United States and Canada 1978–1985.* NIH, Bethesda, MD: U.S. Department of Health and Human Services. (Publication No. 87-2940.)

Shiffman, S. (1982). Relapse following smoking cessation: A situational analysis. *Journal of Consulting and Clinical Psychology, 50*, 71–86.

Shiffman, S. (1984). Coping with temptations to smoke. *Journal of Consulting and Clinical Psychology, 52*, 261–267.

Shiffman, S. (1986). A cluster analytic classification of smoking relapse episodes. *Addictive Behaviors, 11*, 295–307.

Shiffman, S. (in press). Trans-situational consistency in smoking relapse. *Health Psychology.*

Shiffman, S., & Jarvik, M. E. (1987). Situational determinants of coping in smoking relapse crises. *Journal of Applied Social Psychology, 17*, 3–15.

Sjoberg, L., & Johnson, T. (1978). Trying to give up smoking: A study of volitional breakdowns. *Addictive Behaviors, 3*, 149–164.

Supnick, J. A., & Colletti, G. (1984). Relapse coping and problem solving training following treatment for smoking. *Addictive Behaviors, 9*, 401–404.

Swan, G. E., Denk, C. E., Parker, S. D., Carmelli, D., Furze, C. T., & Rosenman, R. H. (1988). Risk factors for late relapse in male and female ex-smokers. *Addictive Behaviors, 13*, 253–266.

Swan, G. E., Parker, S. D., Carmelli, D., Rosenman, R., & Denk, C. E. (1985, August). *The maintenance of smoking cessation as a dynamic process: Multivariate models for males and females.* Paper presented at the meeting of the American Psychological Association, Los Angeles, CA.

U.S. Department of Health and Human Services. (1982). *The health consequences of smoking.* A report of the Surgeon General. *Cancer.* (DHHS Publication No. 82-50-179). Washington, DC: U.S. Government Printing Office.

U.S. National Clearing House for Smoking and Health. (1976). *A survey of health professionals: Smoking and health.* Atlanta, GA: Author.

Wagner, T. J. (1985). Smoking behavior of nurses in western New York. *Nursing Research, 34*, 58–60.

Wewers, M. E. (1988). The role of postcessation factors in tobacco abstinence: Stressful events and coping responses. *Addictive Behaviors, 13*, 297–302.

Wewers, M. E., & Lenz, E. R. (1987). Relapse among ex-smokers: An example of theory derivation. *Advances in Nursing Science, 9*(2), 44–53.

PART II

Research on Nursing Care Delivery

Chapter 5

Home Health Care

VIOLET H. BARKAUSKAS
SCHOOL OF NURSING
THE UNIVERSITY OF MICHIGAN

CONTENTS

Home care has been an organized system of health care in the United States for over 100 years. Home health care was initiated in response to the needs of the poor sick, who had limited choices among options for health care and has endured as an integral component of the American health care system since that time. Professional nurses provided leadership in the initiation and development of home care and continue to be the largest group of professional providers within

The author gratefully acknowledges the contributions of Sawson Majali, M.S.N., R.N., and Betsy Perry, M.P.H., R.N., doctoral students, for assistance in locating and assessing articles for this review.

the field. Additionally, nurses coordinate most of the services of other home health care providers and supervise the work of paraprofessionals, who constitute the largest group of workers within home care. Therefore, much of the research in home care, whether directly related to nursing services or not, has relevance for the practice of nursing.

Three major themes predominate in the research literature related to home health care. First is the evaluation of the efficacy, safety, and cost of home care in comparison with hospital and nursing home care. This theme is especially prominent since the establishment of cost containment through prospective payment by diagnosis related groups (DRGs) because of incentives for early discharge from inpatient acute-care facilities and the resultant home care needs. Similarly, concerns about the costs of caring for a rapidly growing elderly population in residential health care facilities have resulted in research focused on factors influencing long-term hospitalization and mechanisms for the development and provision of long-term home-based services.

The second theme is the use of the home as a convenient location for data collection about health needs and issues and for the testing of interventions with clients. This theme also has become more prominent since prospective payment, possibly because inpatients are less accessible to investigators due to shorter lengths of stay. The studies reflecting this theme are mixed in their relevance to home care practice. Some of these studies are focused on issues fundamental to home health care practice, whereas the content of others is peripheral to the central goals and operations of extant home care practice.

The third theme is the description of the needs of individuals for home-based health-related services and the recipients and providers of such home-based services. The findings of such studies are highly relevant and applicable to home care nursing practice and can serve as bases for future theory development and intervention testing.

The research literature on home care published since 1980 served as the initial source of studies for this review. Citations were obtained from all health-related indexes of printed materials. Additionally, all tables of contents for home care and community health nursing journals since 1980 were hand-searched for relevant articles. All citations appearing to be research reports were located and analyzed for the content and the quality of the reported work. The review was extended by examining reference lists of studies chosen for inclusion, thus selectively extending the search to 1970s publications. The following criteria were used to make the final selection of studies to be cited in the review: (a) content related to nursing practice within home health care and/or on client and intervention phenomena of concern or interest to nurses, and (b) the quality of the research itself. Studies with limited internal and external validity were excluded from the review. However, some studies with moderate methodological limitations were included because of the potential significance of their findings to the field.

Studies selected for inclusion in the review were evaluated by content analysis. The following content outline was established as a result of the analysis and served as the organizing framework for discussion of the literature in this chapter: (a) home health care need and utilization, (b) population groups, (c) selected patient problems, and (d) nurse providers.

A large amount of the published research in the field was on the topic of caregivers. That literature is not included in this review because a complementary review of caregiver research will be published in the *Annual Review of Nursing Research* in a future volume.

HOME HEALTH CARE NEED AND UTILIZATION

As interest in cost containment has increased, research related to home care services utilization has received increased attention. The emphases in such research have been on (a) an understanding of factors affecting need for and use of home care services, (b) the variability of resource consumption among clients receiving home care services, and (c) a comparison of clients using home care with clients using other, usually more expensive and institutional types of care. Because much of the resource allocation in home care is controlled directly or influenced strongly by nurses through referrals and plans of care and because overallocation of nursing services to Medicare clients has been documented (Mundinger, 1983; U.S. General Accounting Office, 1979), utilization research is important to nursing practice.

The research in home care resource need and use has focused heavily on individuals served by the Medicare program. The use of Medicare reimbursement data is logical because of (a) the availability of a national sample for such data, (b) the interest in the impact of

Medicare prospective payment on home care services need and use, (c) the potential application of prospective payment methodologies to a total episode of care, including both in-hospital and posthospital discharge services; and (d) the documented influence of diagnosis related groups on patterns of home care nursing (Kornblatt, Fisher, & MacMillen, 1985). However, focus on the Medicare program limits the study population to the elderly experiencing home care needs resulting from acute illnesses—only one of the multiple client groups within home care systems.

The substantive need for home care services has been documented in several large-scale studies. Soldo (1985) analyzed home care need data collected in conjunction with a national study of 42,000 households that included 110,000 persons. He estimated that 3.2% of all noninstitutionalized persons need home health care at any given point in time. Individuals aged 65 years and older accounted for 58% of all persons classified as needing home care, and approximately 12% of all community-based elderly required home health care of some type.

Given the need of the elderly for home care, it is logical that a substantive proportion of the elderly use home care services. Stone (1986) analyzed data from the National Health Interview Survey collected from January to June, 1985 to determine the elderly's use of community-based services. He found that approximately 2.3% of the elderly aged 65 to 74 years had used home health services in the previous year, and 5.5% of the elderly aged 75 years and over used such services. Berk and Bernstein (1985) determined that the elderly were disproportionately high users of services compared to the rest of the population. Their data from a large-scale study indicated that 4.4% of the elderly used home care over a given time period as compared to 0.7% of persons under age 65 and that 77% of the total number of home care visits were to the elderly although they represented only 43% of the total user population in the study.

In addition to age, a number of factors have been shown to affect home care services use, including the following: type and severity of illness, type of care needs, living arrangements, availability of informal care providers, income level, availability of payment for services, sex, presence and type of recent hospitalization, and geographic area of residence.

Severity of illness, measured by functional limitations and other variables, has been shown to affect home care service use in studies by

Soldo (1985), Stone (1986), and Berk and Bernstein (1985). Individuals reporting limitations in abilities to perform usual or outside activities were more likely to receive home care services than others. Types of diagnoses most frequently represented in home care patients include diseases of the cardiovascular system, diabetes, hypertension, diseases of the nervous system, cancer, and fractures (Berk & Bernstein, 1985; Young & Fisher, 1980). Persons with complex care needs involving treatments and equipment also are more likely to be receiving services (Soldo, 1985).

Living arrangements and availability of informal care providers have been demonstrated to affect use of home care services (Berk & Bernstein, 1985; Soldo, 1985; Stone, 1986). Persons living with others or having informal caregivers available were less likely to be receiving services than others. Logically, persons living with others have greater access to informal care providers for a range of basic general assistance services, for example, shopping, than those living alone.

Berk and Bernstein (1985) found that women and the poor were more likely to use home care sevices than men and the nonpoor. The predominance of women among Medicare patients' use of posthospital care also was noted by Young and Fisher (1980). However, Soldo (1985) concluded that the annual income of caregiving households had only a minor effect on the probability of formal home care services use, and Berk and Bernstein (1985) established that primary sources of payment for home care services were from resources other than clients, clients' families, and private insurance.

Although the majority of home care users have not been hospitalized immediately prior to the receipt of services, recently hospitalized persons are four times more likely to receive home care services than persons not hospitalized (Berk & Bernstein, 1985). Additionally, patients who use posthospital home care reflect a more expensive episode of hospital care (Young & Fisher, 1980).

Geographic area of residence was found to influence both the amount and the types of posthospital care received. Benjamin (1986) studied 1982 Medicare home care services data and demonstrated wide variability in users per 1,000 enrollees and expenditures per user across states within the United States. He found that three fifths of the variation in home care services was explained by seven state characteristics. High use was correlated with low percentage of married persons among the elderly, low percentage of women in the work force, low state tax capacity, high home health agency supply, high percentage of visiting nurse associations among all home health agencies, a large physicians per population ratio, and a high percentage of Title XX funds used for homemaker services for the aged.

Several investigators have explored home care service utilization by studying factors related to the differential use of home care and nursing home services. In an early utilization study limited by a small convenience sample ($N = 44$), McClelland and Kelly (1980) established potential relationships between differential nursing home or home care use and the following variables: sex, presence of a caregiver, functional status, and nursing care requirements. In a more recent study, Kramer, Shaughnessy, and Pettigrew (1985) analyzed case-mix differences between home health and nursing home patients using large random samples drawn from 66 agencies in 12 states. Data analysis revealed that home care patients were younger, had shorter lengths of stay, and were less functionally disabled than nursing home patients. The authors concluded that home care was a cost-effective alternative to nursing home care for patients who did not have significant functional problems.

In addition to understanding the factors influencing use of home care services, investigators also have examined differential use of types and amounts of services received by home care clients. Such data are essential to the establishment of a scientific base for the application of prospective payment mechanisms to the field and for the development of staffing methodologies for home care agencies. A number of agency-based utilization studies were observed in the literature. Day (1984) analyzed 8 years of records ($N = 2,436$ records) from one home care agency and concluded that the amount of home care use is more a function of contextual variables (i.e., referral source, prior source of care, and source payment) than of personal variables (i.e., age, sex, condition, and living arrangments) and that higher intensity of care is associated with likelihood of discharge to self-care for patients receiving short-term home care. In this study, source of payment was the most powerful predictor of both the duration of home care and the intensity of nursing visits: Patients with Medicaid payment reflected longer durations of care with lower intensity of nursing services compared to patients with Medicare, who reflected higher-intensity services of shorter duration.

Pasquale (1987, 1988) conducted a retrospective descriptive study of the demographic characteristics of Medicare home care clients and the scope and the complexity of their health problems using data from 100 randomly selected records in one agency. Results indicated that the typical Medicare home health client was over age 75, female, living alone, relying on informal caregivers, having functional status impairments of at least moderate severity, and experiencing an exacerbation of a chronic medical problem requiring skilled and intermittent care. Additionally, there were more males than females with severe functional impairment being cared for at home, usually by a spouse, possibly indicating that females with severe functional impairments and without available caregivers are likely to be in nursing homes. Pasquale's (1987) conclusions that living arrangements, functional status, and plan of care significantly influenced the consumption of home health care resources are consistent with findings of other cited studies.

Given that patients receiving home care services reflect varying intensities and durations of care, the development of tools to predict resource consumption within home care agencies is logical and has been the focus of two published studies conducted by nurses and a number of additional studies in progress. Peters' (1988) study validating a patient classification scale, the Community Health Intensity Rating Scale, for categorizing patients into one of four levels of nursing care requirements demonstrated significant correlation between estimated levels of nursing care requirements and the actual services provided. In a similar study, Churness, Kleffel, Onodera, and Jacobson (1988) reported the development of a home care patient classification system based on nursing care requirements and historical evidence of the time required for the performance of various nursing assessments and interventions. The tool has enabled nursing staff to classify patients into one of five levels of nursing resource requirements and accurately predict visit duration in 69% of cases.

POPULATION GROUP RESEARCH

Pregnant Women, New Mothers, Infants, and Children

Home care for maternal, infant, and pediatric populations is not new. In the past, the goals of these encounters have been health education for general health promotion. More recently, practice and research have been focused on issues related to the care of individuals at high risk for physical and other health problems and to the home care of sick children. After a review of 24 years of literature on home-based health promotion services for mothers and children, Combs-Orme, Reis, and Ward (1985) concluded that although most studies contained methodological limitations, collective findings indicate that under certain circumstances public health nurses effectively can provide low-income mothers knowledge with the potential to influence parenting practices and long-term infant health outcomes.

Studies of short-term, low-intensity home visiting services to low- or moderate-risk pregnant women and/or new mothers and infants have yielded little evidence of their effectiveness (Barkauskas, 1983). In contrast, evidence of the benefits of long-term, home-based interventions with high-risk populations is increasing. Carpenter et al. (1983) reviewed 7 years of their own research on factors associated with unexpected infant death. Their studies had two thrusts: (a) epidemiological identification of the factors contributing to sudden infant death; and (b) tests of the intervention of frequent, long-term home visiting by health visitors. The authors presented evidence that frequent home visiting to at-risk populations was cost-effective in reducing infant mortality. Another group of researchers (Olds, Henderson, Tatelbaum, & Chamberlin, 1988) demonstrated significant achievements in high school completion, months of employment, and months of postponement of subsequent pregnancies for high-risk women home-visited during pregnancy and for 2 years postpartum. Thus it appears that long-term home interventions can be effective in achieving meaningful outcomes. However, the alleged large-scale cost-effectiveness and feasibility of such interventions is yet to be verified scientifically.

The recent research on home care interventions with pregnant women has been focused on interventions with women at risk for premature labor. Gill and Katz (1986) studied the efficacy of ambulatory tocodynamometers used in conjunction with nursing care for diagnosing preterm labor in 62 at-risk women. Investigators observed that a mean time of 7.5 weeks in utero was gained by infants whose mothers ($n = 29$) were diagnosed in preterm labor. In a similar study (Iams, Johnson, O'Shaughnessy, & West, 1987), a total of 157 women were assigned randomly to one of two treatment groups: (a) a group receiving frequent nursing telephone contact and education regarding symptoms of preterm labor and self-palpation of uterine activity; or (b) a group receiving the same frequent nursing contact by telephone and the use of a mechanical uterine activity monitor. No differences in outcomes were noted between groups, which both experienced beneficial effects. Such studies provide evidence for the value of nursing services in conjunction with high-technology assessment devices and a rationale for further consideration of the relative benefits of technological and nursing assessments.

Various investigators have studied the use of home care as an alternative to longer hospitalization for healthy mothers and their infants as well as for premature infants. James et al. (1987) conducted a quasi-experimental study to determine if early hospital discharge after delivery with home visits by a midwife was as safe as longer hospital stay. The early discharge group ($n = 140$) reflected no increased morbidity and more optimal scores on postpartum adjustment measures than mothers ($n = 156$) discharged later.

Brooten et al. (1986) tested the relative advantages and disadvantages of prolonged inpatient care for premature infants compared with early discharge of such infants. The research involved the random assignment of 79 premature infants to either a control group receiving routine hospital nursery care until they weighed at least 2,200 grams or to an early discharge treatment group in which infants were discharged from the hospital weighing 1,500 grams or less. Early discharge families received instruction, counseling, home visits, and telephone availability from a nurse specialist for 18 months. The two groups did not differ in infants' health outcomes. However, the cost of care for treatment-group infants averaged $18,560 lower than the average cost of care for control-group infants.

Barrera, Cunningham, and Rosenbaum (1986) investigated the effects of long-term home intervention on the development of high-risk infants born prematurely. These researchers discovered that the highest-risk infants and families were more likely to respond favorably to interventions than those at lower risk.

In the cited studies, client self-care at home, supplemented by home nursing care, has been demonstrated to be a safe, cost-effective alternative to hospitalization or extended hospitalization for healthy mothers and infants as well as for high-risk infants. However, in all of the cited studies investigators provided limited information regarding the content of home-based nursing interventions. Clearly, research about the nature of the interventions themselves and comparisons among various types of and approaches to home interventions is indicated.

The research on home care of children beyond infancy has been focused on (a) the safety of home care for children discharged with complex treatments or for severely disabled, chronically ill children;

(b) the abilities of family members to care for such children at home; and (c) the use of home care as a parent substitute for working parents with mildly ill children needing to stay home from school. Burr, Guyer, Todres, Abrahams, and Chiodo (1983) and Bosch and Cuyler (1987) explored issues related to families' abilities to care for ventilator-dependent children ($N = 6$) and children with tracheostomies ($N = 16$). In both studies investigators documented the abilities of selected parents and other caregivers to manage technologically complex home care safely with professional assistance and presented evidence that home care is beneficial in a variety of dimensions. Additionally, Burr et al. (1983) documented the cost saving of home care for such children when costs were compared with hospital care. Similarly, Donati, Guenette, and Auerbach (1987) were able to demonstrate comparable effectiveness between home and hospital treatment for patients with exacerbations of pulmonary disease due to cystic fibrosis, and significantly lower costs for home care.

Given the potential benefits of home care for seriously and chronically ill children, research on the abilities of their family caregivers and their responses to nursing interventions is very relevant. Athreya and McCormick (1987) studied the impact of severely handicapped children on their families ($N = 483$) and determined that significant predictors of family impact included the number of children's activities of daily living limited by health and the educational attainment of the mother. Needs of families for home care assistance are not restricted to situations in which children are seriously ill. In separate studies in the United States and the United Kingdom, Andrews, Nuttall, and Nielson (1987) and Emery, Waite, Carpenter, Limerick, and Blake (1985) documented that the use of a common, high-technology monitoring device, the apnea monitor, could result in a number of educational, technical, safety, and emotional problems within families of infants using the device but that home nursing services could assist parents in managing the problems.

Marshall (1987) examined the adequacy of the preparation for hospital discharge and the subsequent community care received by the families ($N = 20$) of infants recently discharged from a neonatal surgical unit in the United Kingdom. Study findings indicated that families generally received adequate teaching regarding specialized procedures but minimal preparation in psychological and social domains from the surgical unit staff. Community services were found to vary greatly, and parents generally were dissatisfied with the technical competence of community services staffs. Similar dissatisfactions with community services were noted by mothers of severely mentally handicapped schoolchildren (Ayer, 1984).

Kun and Warburton (1987) studied parents' ($N = 60$) knowledge of home care treatments during telephone interviews conducted 48 hours after hospital discharge. Knowledge deficits were observed in parents whose children required complex single procedures or multiple procedures. However, knowledge deficits were not correlated significantly with subsequent hospitalizations in this study.

Research about the adequacy of home care of mildly ill children enrolled in day care centers as an alternative arrangement for working parents was conducted by Chang, Kelso, Harris, and Jordan (1981). Home care was provided by trained home workers, and children were assigned randomly to receive a combination of worker and parent care ($n = 23$) or parent care alone ($n = 46$). Interestingly, episodes of illness in children cared for by trained home workers had slightly shorter durations and less severe courses when compared with episodes of illness in children cared for by parents only.

The Elderly

Most of the research on home care services for the elderly has been focused on services for ill or functionally compromised elderly. However, the benefits of preventive home care services for the elderly were explored in one located study. Hendriksen, Lund, and Stromgard (1984) studied the health services utilization and health of over 500 randomly selected subjects aged 75 years or older living in Denmark. Approximately half of the group received nurse home visits directed at enhancing self-care and scheduled at intervals of at least one visit every 3 months for a duration of 1½ years. Significant reduction in numbers of hospital admissions, numbers of emergency medical calls, and deaths were noted in the treatment group. Calculation of estimated costs of interventions and savings provided strong evidence for the cost-effectiveness of preventive interventions for the elderly.

Numerous studies have been focused on the home health care needs of and the outcomes of home care services on sick and frail elderly with emphases on the costs and benefits of maintaining individuals in their homes and preventing long-term hospitalizations. The findings among these studies are inconsistent, possibly due to unknown variations among subjects and interventions. In a New York-based study Brickner et al. (1976) demonstrated that home care for homebound elderly persons could be less expensive than institutional care for many elderly persons. In a later study of statewide implementation to maintain elderly Medicaid patients in their homes in New York State, Gaumer et al. (1986) concluded that the program had been successful in reducing nursing home admissions but that cost savings varied by patients' geographic residence.

In contrast, findings from a Chicago-based study in which the outcomes of a treatment group ($n = 157$) of frail elderly receiving multidisciplinary home care for 48 months were compared with those of a comparison group ($n = 156$) included a significantly lower risk of permanent admission to sheltered and intermediate-level nursing homes in the treatment group, no between-group differences in admissions to hospitals and skilled-level nursing facilities, but significantly more in-hospital days and 25% higher costs in the treatment group (Hughes, Cordray, & Spiker, 1984; Hughes, Manheim, Edelman, & Conrad, 1987). However, significant quality of life benefits were noted in the treatment group.

Zimmer, Groth-Juncker, and McCusker (1985) randomly assigned homebound, terminally ill elderly to team care or routine care to determine the effectiveness of a home care team approach. The team included a physician, a nurse practitioner, and a social worker. Findings indicated that team patients ($n = 81$) had fewer hospitalizations, nursing home admissions, and outpatient visits than controls ($n = 75$). Functional abilities of team patients did not differ from controls, and the total costs of care did not differ between groups. Team patients expressed significantly higher satisfaction with health care received.

A British study (Currie et al., 1980) of the feasibility and efficacy of caring for acutely and subacutely ill elderly patients at home was conducted through a scheme of augmented home care as an alternative to hospitalization in an acute-care facility. The findings from the study, involving 37 patients, indicated that functional recovery was more rapid at home than in the hospital and that home care was feasible and acceptable to patients. Findings from another British study (Gibbens et al., 1982) of augmented home nursing as an alternative to hospital care for chronically ill elderly ($N = 24$) contained implications that (a) augmented home care may be more suitable and less expensive than hospital care if nighttime supervision is not needed or if such supervision can be provided informally and (b) augmented home care is preferable to long-stay hospital care. In another study of alternative sources of care, Hu, Huang, and Cartwright (1986) compared the costs of caring for senile, demented elderly individuals at home ($n = 25$) with care in a nursing home ($n = 19$). Costs of home care were approximately half of the costs of nursing home care.

Capitman (1986) conducted a national evaluation of five community-oriented, long-term care projects funded by the Health Care Financing Administration. The innovative intervention tested in the majority of these projects was augmentation of home care services. Although two of these projects served persons under age 65, the majority of clients were elderly, and at least one fifth of the participants across projects were age 85 or older. Care provided through these demonstration projects had no effect on acute-care facility use, and only one of the projects demonstrated significantly fewer nursing home days for treatment groups than for comparison groups. Capitman concluded that neither functional status nor demographic variables clearly predicted use of acute-care facilities or nursing homes for the studied populations. Similar conclusions about the inconsistency of evidence for the effectiveness of expanded home care programs were made by Hughes (1985).

SELECTED PATIENT PROBLEMS

Research has been conducted on home care services related to the following patient needs and problems: intravenous infusions, respiratory therapy, hypertension, arthritis, cancer, cerebrovascular accidents, myocardial infarction, diabetes, decubitus ulcers, and psychiatric problems. The primary focus of most of these studies has been the exploration of the safety and acceptability of home care as an alternative site for care. Secondary foci have been tertiary prevention for individuals already compromised by chronic illness and tests of new therapies for the management of chronic problems.

Two groups of researchers (Nieweg, Greidanus, & de Vries, 1987; Stiver, Trosky, Cote, & Oruck, 1982) studied the feasibility and safety of the continuation of intravenous therapy with nursing services from an inpatient setting in the home. Findings from both studies indicated that home care was as safe as continuous hospital care for carefully selected patients.

Patients with respiratory conditions have been the focus of several studies. The Medical Research Council Working Party (1981) noted the long-term benefits of decreased mortality and slowing of deterioration for patients with chronic obstructive chest diseases by use of home oxygen therapy. Make and Gilmartin (1986) reviewed the literature regarding home care for ventilator-dependent individuals. These authors concluded that home ventilator therapy is safe and effective but that the management of the practice is inconsistent and in need of additional study. A team of investigators (Cockcroft et al., 1987; Heslop & Bagnall, 1988) evaluated the benefits of home nursing services to patients with disabling chest diseases. The study sample included 75 patients with chronic chest diseases who were randomly assigned to experimental ($n = 42$) or control groups ($n = 33$). Experimental group patients received home visiting services from nurses and demonstrated significant improvement in knowledge about their conditions. However, no or only moderately positive differences between groups were noted in quality of life measures and death rates. The home-visited group experienced fewer but longer hospitalizations than the control group, possibly reflecting admissions for only severe illnesses in the home-visited group.

Two studies on the treatment of pressure ulcers are examples of clinically relevant research on home care nursing interventions. Boykin and Winland-Brown (1986) compared treatment of pressure sores ($n = 5$ subjects) with providone-iodine in one agency with hydrocolloid occlusive dressings ($n = 6$ subjects) in a second agency, and Sebern (1986) tested the efficacy and cost of treating pressure ulcers with a new moisture vapor permeable dressing. In both studies significant improvements in healing were noted, and the costs of care were lower for clients receiving experimental treatments.

Hopper, Miller, Birge, and Swift (1984) conducted a study of the effects of home health aide services on the health and health services utilization of low-income diabetic patients. Subjects using aide services ($n = 44$) showed significant increase in keeping eye clinic appointments as well as reduction in fasting blood sugar levels.

Several British researchers (Hill, Hampton, & Mitchell, 1978, 1979) conducted a 4-year randomized trial comparing home versus hospital management of patients with suspected myocardial infarction. A total of 364 patients were assigned randomly to either home or hospital management of their acute myocardial infarction after intensive emergency care in the home. A 6-week follow-up of all study patients indicated that mortality was similar between groups. Other studies contained evidence for various other home-based interventions for persons suspected of having myocardial infarctions or diagnosed with the problem (Adgey & Crampton, 1981; Bell, Thomas, Isaacson, Snell, & Holt, 1982; Moore et al., 1986).

Various issues related to the home care of patients after cerebrovascular accidents have been investigated. Legh-Smith, Wade, and Langton-Hewer (1986) explored the use of community services by 492 patients 1 year after their cerebrovascular accidents. A total of 38% of the subjects ($n = 143$) received community-based services, the most common of which were district nursing (73 subjects), home help (73 subjects), day centers (42 subjects), and home-delivered meals (30 subjects). Anderson, Anderson, and Kottke (1977) conducted a retrospective study of stroke patients after discharge from an inpatient rehabilitation program. The investigators concluded that improvements in functional status resulting from rehabilitation were maintained and continued after discharge. Independent variables correlating with positive rehabilitation variables included living at home rather than in a nursing home and having an accepting attitude. Wade, Langton-Hewer, Skilbeck, Bainton, and Burns-Cox (1985) conducted a large controlled trial of augmented home care for 6 months after a cerebrovascular accident ($N = 857$ patients). As in other trials of home care augmentation, this one demonstrated few differences between subjects receiving additional services and those who selectively used existing home care services.

The home care needs of terminally ill cancer patients and the effect of home care on the costs of care and the well-being of patients and families have been explored in a number of studies. Googe and Varricchio (1981) conducted a small pilot study to describe the home care needs of cancer patients ($N = 15$) and their families. The investigators determined that most needs of daily living were met by family members, with needs requiring special skills shared between family members and home care nurses. The problems frequently identified by patients included equipment, transportation, pain management, elimination, bathing, eating, ambulation, special skills, sleep, and information about home care. The problems of family members included need for household help, need for help with shopping, additional expenses due to patient care, loss of sleep, unsatisfactory health, need for help in emergency situations, need for information about home care, and interruption in family eating schedule. Another exploratory, descriptive study by Pringle and Taylor (1984) focused on the needs of terminally ill patients and the home care services provided to them. Pain, loss of appetite, sleep disturbances, and constipation were the most frequently reported symptoms.

Vinciguerra and associates (Vinciguerra, Degnan, Budman, et al., 1986; Vinciguerra, Degnan, Sciortino, et al., 1986) conducted a prospective study of the comparative costs and other outcomes of hospital and home care of terminally ill cancer patients. Subjects were assigned to home or hospital treatment based on geographic location; home care was provided by a team of health professionals, including a nurse. The health benefits of home care included decreased narcotic analgesia needs, decreased hospitalization, decreased hospital length of stay, and improved survival. Other investigators (McCusker & Stoddard, 1987) used a quasi-experimental, retrospective design to determine if an expanded program of home care for terminally ill patients provided during the last month of life would reduce hospital utilization and the total costs of care during this time. Data were derived from tumor registries and insurance company claims. Patients using home care demonstrated significant reduction in hospital care days and the mean per diem cost of hospitalization and less variability in total costs of care when compared to nonusers of home care.

Liang et al. (1984) explored the effectiveness of comprehensive rehabilitation services for elderly homebound patients with arthritis and orthopedic disability. Patients were recruited from the caseloads of home care agencies, and the services provided through the study were supplementary to those provided by the home care agencies. Subjects were assigned randomly to treatment and control groups in a crossover design, enabling all subjects to receive the treatment prior to the end of the study. Services were provided by physical therapists to 57 subjects, and functional ability, institutionalization, and contentment outcomes were measured. Although some patients achieved substantial benefit per anecdotal reports, findings indicated no significant differences between treatment and control groups after the first phase of the study and from admission to the end of the study.

Several pilot studies regarding the efficacy of home care with psychiatric patients as an alternative or as a supplement to hospital care have been published (Heymann & Stanton, 1977; Pai & Nagarajaiah, 1982). Specific data about outcomes were not reported for these studies, but the authors provided anecdotal evidence supporting the efficacy of home nursing care in achieving improved functioning and decreased hospitalization for treatment groups. Paykel, Mangen, Griffith, and Burns (1982) conducted a study of 71 neurotic outpatients who were assigned randomly to routine treatment or to home care from community psychiatric nurses. Home nursing care compared very favorably with routine clinic care in outcomes after 18 months of service.

The ability of hypertensive patients to assume primary responsibility for providing self-care and monitoring the results of such has been explored by several investigators who consistently have concluded that patients can be taught to measure blood pressure at home accurately (Cottier, Julius, Gajendragadkar, & Schork, 1982; Fitzgerald et al., 1985). In another study (Earp, Ory, & Strogatz, 1982) of hypertension control, subjects were assigned randomly to one of two treatment groups or a control group. Subjects in the first treatment group ($n = 99$) received home visits and family members were involved actively in their care; subjects in the second treatment group ($n = 56$) received home visits from nurses and pharmacists; and the control group ($n = 63$) received routine care. After 1 year of intervention, the groups demonstrated no statistical differences for outcome variables. However, after 2 years the treatment groups demonstrated significantly lower percentages of individuals with uncontrolled diastolic blood pressures. Subjects in this study received an average of approximately five visits over 18 months.

NURSE PROVIDERS

A small amount of research has been conducted about home care nurses. Currently an estimated 40% of the 101,000 nurses working in community health nursing are practicing home health care in the estimated total of 10,000 certified and noncertified home care agencies in the United States (Spiegel, 1987; U.S. Department of Health and Human Services, 1988), and an unknown number of nurses provide home care through public health departments and hospital-based home care programs. These data represent a 33% increase in the number of nurses and a 95% increase in the number of Medicare-certified agencies since 1980 (Spiegel, 1987; U.S. Department of Health and Human Services, 1988).

The foci of research on home health care nurses have been identification of job stresses and assessments of nurses' competence. Stanek (1987) conducted a small study comparing job stresses between skilled nursing facility nurses and home health care nurses. The primary stresses identified by home care nurses were paperwork, case overload, and job performance responsibilities. Overall, home care nurses reflected low to moderate levels of burnout on standardized instruments.

Exploration of the competencies of home care nurses is logical given the isolated nature of their practice. Home care nurses rarely observe other nurses or professionals in their daily encounters with patients and families. The work of home care nurses with maternal and child health client groups was explored in two studies. Schulze and Koerner (1987) measured the attitudes toward maternal and child health care responsibilities of 122 community health nurses from nine voluntary nonprofit agencies in one state. Study findings revealed that 73% of community-based nurses in the sample perceived a deficit of knowledge for the care of such clients. Von Windeguth, Urbano, Hayes, and Martyn (1988) conducted a retrospective analysis of 30 records of families with infants at risk for developmental disabilities to determine the reflected competencies of the nurses providing services. Data collected from only one agency indicated that assessments of parent–infant interaction and the animate environment were not documented in a majority of the records reviewed. However, the nurses characteristically assessed infants for previously established biological risks.

Bernal and Froman (1987) conducted a study of the confidence of community health nurses in caring for ethnically diverse populations. The sample included 190 respondents (a 38% response rate) from a variety of community health nursing agencies, including home care agencies, in Connecticut. Findings indicated that nurses felt moderate to low confidence in caring for clients from black, Puerto Rican, and Southeast Asian ethnic backgrounds.

Clarke, Goggin, Webber-Jones, Vacek, and Aderholdt (1986) evaluated the effectiveness of an educational program in respiratory assessment given to 34 nurses in five rural home care agencies in Vermont. Study findings indicated that learners' abilities in inspection, palpation, and percussion increased significantly after 10 collaborative training visits and that the learning was maintained at a 6-month postttest. However, competency with auscultation occurred after 20 collaborative visits and regressed to preinstruction levels at the 6-month posttest.

SYNTHESIS

The foci of home care research reflect a collage of the multiple and diverse client groups served by professional nurses. Much of the cited research in home care could easily have been included in reviews of studies focused on a particular client group, for example, the elderly, or a particular problem, for example, intravenous infusion. However, the consistency of findings across client groups and problems is evidence of the probable existence of a unique treatment effect for home care intervention.

The research in home care contains documentation of the need for home care services and their effectiveness across diverse population groups, including patients as well as their caregivers. Evidence exists that the ill elderly will continue to be the major client group for home care services. However, researchers have documented the relevance and effectiveness of home-based preventive, acute-care, and chronic-care services for individuals across the life span.

Through utilization studies investigators have sought to differentiate the users of home care services from nonusers or users of potentially more expensive sources of care, for example nursing homes, and to determine factors associated with the amount of home care services received. Research has focused primarily on the elderly because of their high service use and because of the availability of utilization data from the Medicare program. Findings across utilization studies have been generally consistent, with the following factors demonstrating influence on the use of home care services: geographic residence, functional status, sex, economic situation, recent medical history, and living arrangements (Benjamin, 1986; Berk & Bernstein, 1985). Once a patient is admitted to services, the amount of care received is affected by treatment needs, referral source, source of care, type of payment, and living arrangements (Ballard & McNamara, 1983; Day, 1984; Pasquale, 1987). Nursing home patients have been shown to differ from home care patients in the dimensions of age and functional status, with nursing home patients generally being significantly older and more disabled (Kramer et al., 1985).

Research on home care for disease prevention and health maintenance goals has demonstrated consistently that long-term home care provided to high-risk clients can be effective in decreasing risk and preventing untoward outcomes for significant percentages of individuals, whereas there is no evidence of effectiveness of low-intensity home care with low-risk populations. However, it can be argued that intervention with high-risk individuals is really a form of secondary prevention, or early treatment, rather than primary prevention. These conclusions are consistent with those of reviews by Combs-Orme et al. (1985), Carpenter et al. (1983), and Halpern (1986).

The high cost of institutional care and emphasis on cost containment have stimulated experimentation in early discharge from acute-care facilities, as well as avoidance of admission to them. The following conclusions can be derived from the review of the studies on use of the home as an alternative site for individuals experiencing acute-care needs, the terminally ill, and children with serious chronic illnesses:

1. A variety of treatments and care regimens can be provided safely at home by formal and informal caregivers and by the patients themselves.
2. In addition to being less expensive than hospital care, home care is usually more acceptable to patients and families.
3. Patients and families often have unmet needs for information, guidance, and assistance with coping strategies during their transition from acute-care facilities to home.

The literature is extensive and rich in supporting these conclusions across population groups. Examples include James et al. (1987) for maternity and infant patients; Brooten et al. (1986) for premature infants; Burr et al. (1983), Bosch and Cuyler (1987), and Marshall (1987) for severely ill children with ventilators, tracheostomies, and other care needs; Martinson et al. (1986) for terminally ill children; Currie et al. (1980) for acutely ill elderly; Stiver et al. (1982) for intravenous antibiotic therapy; Nieweg et al. (1987) for vascular access pump therapy; Make and Gilmartin (1986) for ventilator-dependent persons; Cockcroft et al. (1987) and Heslop and Bagnall (1988) for patients with disabling chest diseases; Adgey and Crampton (1981), Bell et al. (1982), and Hill et al. (1978, 1979) for patients with myocardial infarction; Vinciguerra, Degnan, Budman, et al. (1986), Vinciguerra, Degnan, Sciortino, et al. (1986), and McCusker and Stoddard (1987) for terminally ill adults; and Earp et al. (1982) for hypertension management. Clearly, the evidence that selected patients and families can manage care adequately at home with assistance from the home care system is compelling. However, it must be noted that subjects across studies were chosen carefully for their abilities to participate in care, and findings from many studies may not be generalizable to all members of the target populations.

Findings across studies of the effectiveness of home-based health maintenance care to chronically ill individuals are inconsistent, probably because of varying samples and diverse measurement approaches represented across studies. Also, the predominant dependent variable of interest in these studies has been cost containment through prevention of both acute-care and long-term care hospitalization, with some, but relatively little, attention to quality of life and other dependent variables. Two well-controlled studies have demonstrated contradictory findings about the cost-effectiveness of special home care services, that is, lack of cost-effectiveness in Hughes et al. (1984, 1987) and cost-effectiveness in Zimmer et al. (1985). These observations are consistent with the conclusions of other reviews on this subject (Capitman, 1986; Gaumer et al., 1986; Hedrick & Inui, 1986; Hughes, 1985). Likewise, studies focused on the benefits of supplemental home care services to patients experiencing care needs resultant from either acute or chronic problems have yielded little evidence of the benefits of augmented home care services.

THEORETICAL, METHODOLOGICAL, AND ANALYTICAL ISSUES

In the majority of studies cited, investigators have paid little or no attention to the presentation of theoretical explanations for study problems, questions, and hypotheses. Even in cases in which the interventions were provided by specially trained personnel hired and supervised by project staffs, home care was treated as a known commodity, and little attempt was made to establish theoretical rationales for the variables studied, the interventions provided, or the outcomes achieved. This lack of a theoretical base for the research in the field is limiting, especially when comparisons among studies are attempted. One exception to this observation is an exploratory study by King, Figge, and Harman (1986) in which relationships among the theoretical constructs of coping at home after recent hospitalization, certainty/uncertainty about current circumstances, perceptions about health, and satisfaction with care were proposed and explored.

The reviewed studies represent diverse methodological approaches, including descriptive studies with small sample sizes, quasi-experimental studies with self-selected intervention groups or poorly controlled comparison groups, well-controlled experiments with longitudinal follow-up of subjects, and broad-based population surveys with very large sample sizes. The measurement tools used in home care research have reflected the broad scope of types of tools used in research and have varied among the studies. The field does not have consistent approaches for measurement of most critical variables of interest. The predominant dependent variables in most of the intervention studies were economic. This focus has been practical and rational. However, given the evidence that home care can be cost-effective for many patient groups, it would seem that work directed to the identification and measurement of other relevant types of variables, for example, health, function, and comfort, is indicated for future research. In most instances, tools were developed for the specific studies, and data about pilot testing, validity, or reliability were not presented.

The field reflects almost no replication of methods; therefore, findings can be applied only with great caution. Moreover, most of the intervention studies were conducted in only one agency or health care system and used the staff in that agency or a small project staff as the providers of services, thus limiting the generalizability of findings.

Another factor limiting generalizability and supporting the need for replication is the lack of control for or measurement of additional home care and health care services received by study subjects. In a number of studies there is indication that both control as well as treatment subjects received an unspecified number of home care and other health care services that could have affected study findings.

Findings of studies focused on the abilities of patients and/or caregivers to implement complex therapies or assessments at home successfully must be applied cautiously because of the biases in subject selection. In most of the studies in which a complex treatment was transferred to home care in lieu of extended hospitalization, study methods indicated that patients and caregivers were selected carefully. More research on factors affecting the abilities of general home care populations is indicated. A recent exploratory study by Stiller (1988) contained interesting insights into theoretical and methodological approaches to the investigation of the issues related to patients' successes and difficulties with high-technology home care.

In most studies data were analyzed using simple statistical methods, although complex multivariate analytical approaches were used in some studies. Data analysis techniques generally have been appropriate to the questions and the amounts and types of data obtained. Serious omissions in presentations of data were power analyses, assessment of pretreatment equivalence, and assessments of withdrawals after random assignment.

NURSING INTERVENTIONS IN HOME CARE

A proposition that most home care research is potentially relevant to nursing because of nursing's centrality to the field was made in the introduction to this chapter. As more types and amounts of health care are transferred from institutions, the nurse roles in home care will expand, and the development of relevant research will be critical to the development of nursing practice within the field. However, much of the reviewed research, although relevant to home care nursing, has neither been conducted by nurses nor has included specific discussion of nursing participation.

Although the findings about nursing practice in home care are sparse, their consistency is worthy of note and comment. Nursing was identified as a major portion of the intervention in the methodologically strongest of the studies cited. However, even in the strong studies, the theoretical bases for nursing intervention were not discussed, and the nursing interventions generally were described as telephone contacts and home visits (e.g., Carpenter et al., 1983; Gill & Katz, 1986; Hendriksen et al., 1984; Iams et al., 1987). Given that a number of the studies were designed using specially hired and oriented nurses as the care providers, major opportunities for the measurement of specific nursing interventions within encounters were lost. Only in the studies by Brooten et al. (1986), Cockcroft et al. (1987), and Olds et al. (1988) were attempts made to structure the foci and content of the nursing encounters, but in none of these studies were the specific interventions provided within nursing encounters reported.

In the studies describing the intended foci and content of nursing encounters, the predominant intervention strategy themes were assessment, education, encouragement, counseling, and support. Although these studies provided evidence for the effectiveness of home care nursing with high-risk populations, the theoretical bases of practice were not developed to the extent possible because of unspecified assumptions about the dynamics of nurse–patient encounters and the lack of documentation of the encounters themselves beyond the counting of encounters and the time represented by them.

FUTURE DIRECTIONS

One major knowledge deficit in the field is lack of theoretical propositions to support nursing practice in the field. Home care fits into the broad specialty of community health nursing, which claims numerous conceptual bases but no well-developed, dynamic, theoretical base to explain the dynamics of nurse–client encounters and to link those dynamics with changes in clients' conditions.

One major conceptual question relates to the meaning of "home" beyond the setting for care. Underlying implicit assumptions embedded in the research and the general professional literature on home care are that "home" connotes more than setting—that, additionally, the concept reflects notions such as resource, environment, support, self-care, and so on. Therefore, the exploration of these notions is important to understanding the dynamics of patient–nurse encounters in home care and identification of appropriate outcome measures for clinical trials.

The major focus on economic outcome measures has been relevant to the current cost-containment paradigm in health services research. However, such focus is very narrow, and work on the identification of a more holistic array of outcome variables for home care research is timely, given projected emphases on quality assessment in health services research. Moreover, although the home has proven to be a cost-effective site for acute care as an alternative site to hospital care, home care may not be cost-effective in comparison to other approaches to care, for example, ambulatory clinic care or group care. Expansion of the pool of outcome variables would enable creative comparisons among the assets and liabilities of various potential settings for care across client groups.

The extant research on home care has produced a large data base on home care clients and their needs and problems. However, little is known about the components and dynamics of home-based nursing interventions. Fundamental to the formulation of practice theories in the field is the development of methods for measuring and classifying home care services to clients and for describing the patterns of such services. Some instrument development for the description of services has begun, and the preliminary findings are promising (Churness et al., 1988; Garrard, Dowd, Dorsey, & Shapiro, 1987; Martin, 1988; Peters, 1988; Storfjell, 1987), but all tools need substantive validity and reliability assessment.

The strength of the research findings relating to interventions with high-risk individuals is justification for the continuation of the research related to the identification of these groups and the testing of preventive interventions with them. Given the current trends toward enhancing health promotion through self-care and prevention and the avoidance of the use of inpatient services, this research is relevant as well as marketable.

This review supports the importance of home care and the need for future research into multiple aspects of home care clients, providers, and services to assure scientific and responsible developments of the field. Nurses have been and are increasingly essential and central to the provision of home care services and are making substantive contributions to the development of the scientific base for the field.

REFERENCES

Adgey, A. A. J., & Crampton, R. S. (1981). Hospital or home for acute myocardial infarction: Another look at whether or not we should bother to care. *American Heart Journal, 102*, 473–477.

Anderson, E., Anderson, T. P., & Kottke, F. J. (1977). Stroke rehabilitation: Maintenance of achieved gains. *Archives of Physical Medicine and Rehabilitation, 58*, 345–352.

Andrews, M. M., Nuttall, P. R., & Nielson, D. W. (1987). Home apnea monitoring in the Intermountain West. *Journal of Pediatric Health Care, 1*, 255–260.

Athreya, B. H., & McCormick, M. C. (1987). Impact of chronic illness on families. *Rheumatic Disease Clinics of North America, 13*, 123–131.

Ayer, S. (1984). Community care: Failure of professionals to meet family needs. *Child: Care, Health and Development, 10*, 127–140.

Ballard, S., & McNamara, R. (1983). Quantifying nursing needs in home health care. *Nursing Research, 32*, 236–241.

Barkauskas, V. H. (1983). Effectiveness of public health nurse home visits to primiparous mothers and their infants. *American Journal of Public Health, 73*, 573–580.

Barrera, M. E., Cunningham, C. E., & Rosenbaum, P. L. (1986). Low birth weight and home intervention strategies: Preterm infants. *Journal of Developmental and Behavioral Pediatrics, 7*, 361–366.

Bell, J. A., Thomas, J. M., Isaacson, J. R., Snell, N. J. C., & Holt, D. W. (1982). A trial of prophylactic mexiletine in home coronary care. *British Heart Journal, 48,* 285–290.

Benjamin, A. E. (1986). Determinants of state variations in home health utilization and expenditures under Medicare. *Medical Care, 24,* 535–547.

Berk, M. L., & Bernstein, A. (1985). Use of home health services: Some findings from the National Medical Care Expenditure Survey. *Home Health Care Services Quarterly, 6*(1), 13–23.

Bernal, H., & Froman, R. (1987). The confidence of community health nurses in caring for ethnically diverse populations. *Image: Journal of Nursing Scholarship, 19,* 201–203.

Bosch, J. D., & Cuyler, J. P. (1987). Home care of the pediatric tracheostomy: Our experience. *The Journal of Otolaryngology, 16,* 120–122.

Boykin, A., & Winland-Brown, J. (1986). Pressure sores: Nursing management. *Journal of Gerontological Nursing, 12*(12), 17–21.

Brickner, P. W., Janeski, J. F., Rich, G., Duque, T., Starita, L., LaRocco, R., Flannery, T., & Werlin, S. (1976). Home maintenance for the homebound aged. *The Gerontologist, 16,* 25–29.

Brooten, D., Kumar, S., Brown, L. P., Butts, P., Finkler, S. A., Bakewell-Sachs, S., Gibbons, A., & Delivoria-Papadopoulos, M. (1986). A randomized clinical trial of early hospital discharge and home follow-up of very-low-birth-weight infants. *New England Journal of Medicine, 315,* 934–939.

Burr, B. H., Guyer, B., Todres, I. D., Abrahams, B., & Chiodo, T. (1983). Home care for children on respirators. *New England Journal of Medicine, 309,* 1319–1323.

Capitman, J. A. (1986). Community-based long-term care models, target groups, and impacts on service use. *The Gerontologist, 26,* 389–397.

Carpenter, R. G., Gardner, A., Jepsen, M., Taylor, E. M., Salvin, A., Sunderland, R., Emery, J. L., Pursall, E., & Roe, J. (1983). Prevention of unexpected infant death: Evaluation of the first seven years of the Sheffield Intervention Programme. *The Lancet, 1*(8327), 723–727.

Chang, A., Kelso, G., Harris, M., & Jordan, A. (1981). Care of mildly ill children enrolled in day care centers: Management by parents and by trained home workers. *The Western Journal of Medicine, 134,* 181–185.

Churness, V. H., Kleffel, D., Onodera, M. L., & Jacobson, J. (1988). Reliability and validity testing of a home health patient classification system. *Public Health Nursing, 5,* 135–139.

Clarke, J. H., Goggin, J. E., Webber-Jones, J. E., Vacek, P. M., & Aderholdt, S. (1986). Educating rural home health care nurses in respiratory assessment: An evaluation study. *Public Health Nursing, 3,* 101–110.

Cockcroft, A., Bagnall, P., Heslop, A., Andersson, N., Heaton, R., Batstone, J., Allen, J., Spencer, P., & Guz, A. (1987). Controlled trial of respiratory health worker visiting patients with chronic respiratory disability. *British Medical Journal, 294,* 225–228.

Combs-Orme, T., Reis, J., & Ward, L. D. (1985). Effectiveness of home visits by public health nurses in maternal and child health: An empirical review. *Public Health Reports, 100,* 490–499.

Cottier, C., Julius, S., Gajendragadkar, S. V., & Schork, M. A. (1982).

Usefulness of home BP determination in treating borderline hypertension. *Journal of American Medical Association, 248,* 555–558.

Currie, C. T., Burley, L. E., Doull, C., Ravetz, C., Smith, R. G., & Williamson, J. (1980). A scheme of augmented home care for acutely and subacutely ill elderly patients: Report on pilot study. *Age and Aging, 9,* 173–180.

Day, S. R. (1984). Measuring utilization and impact of home care services: A systems model approach for cost-effectiveness. *Home Health Care Services Quarterly, 5*(2), 5–24.

Donati, M. A., Guenette, G., & Auerbach, H. (1987). Prospective controlled study of home and hospital therapy of cystic fibrosis pulmonary disease. *Journal of Pediatrics, 111,* 28–33.

Earp, J. L., Ory, M. G., & Strogatz, D. S. (1982). The effects of family involvement and practitioner home visits on the control of hypertension. *American Journal of Public Health, 72,* 1146–1153.

Emery, J. L., Waite, A. J., Carpenter, R. G., Limerick, S. R., & Blake, D. (1985). Apnea monitors compared with weighing scales for siblings after cot death. *Archives of Diseases of Children, 60,* 1055–1060.

Fitzgerald, D. J., O'Callaghan, W. G., O'Brien, E., Johnson, H., Mulcahy, R., & Hickey, N. (1985). Home recording of blood pressure in the management of hypertension. *Irish Medical Journal, 78,* 216–218.

Garrard, J., Down, B. E., Dorsey, B., & Shapiro, J. (1987). A checklist to assess the need for home health care: Instrument development and validation. *Public Health Nursing, 4,* 212–218.

Gaumer, G. L., Birnbaum, H., Pratter, F., Burke, R., Franklin, S., & Ellingson-Otto, K. (1986). Impact of the New York Long-Term Home Health Care Program. *Medical Care, 24,* 641–653.

Gibbens, F. J., Lee, M., Davison, P. R., O'Sullivan, P., Hutchinson, M., Murphy, D. R., & Ugwu, C. N. (1982). Augmented home nursing as an alternative to hospital care for chronic elderly invalids. *British Medical Journal, 284,* 330–333.

Gill, P. J., & Katz, M. (1986). Early detection of preterm labor: Ambulatory home monitoring of uterine activity. *Journal of Gynecologic and Neonatal Nursing, 15,* 439–442.

Googe, M. C., & Varricchio, C. G. (1981). A pilot investigation of home health care needs of cancer patients and their families. *Oncology Nursing Forum, 8*(4) 24–28.

Halpern, R. (1986). Home based early intervention: Dimensions of current practice. *Child Welfare, 65,* 387–398.

Hedrick, S. C., & Inui, T. S. (1986). The effectiveness and cost of home care: An information synthesis. *Health Services Research, 20,* 851–880.

Hendriksen, C., Lund, E., & Stromgard, E. (1984). Consequences of assessment and intervention among elderly people: A three year randomized controlled trial. *British Medical Journal, 289,* 1522–1524.

Heslop, A. P., & Bagnall, P. (1988). A study to evaluate the intervention of a nurse visiting patients with disabling chest disease in the community. *Journal of Advanced Nursing, 13,* 71–77.

Heymann, G. M., & Stanton, L. M. (1977). A pilot study to evaluate visiting nurses' services to chronic psychiatric patients. *Hospital and Community Psychiatry, 28*(2), 97, 101.

Hill, J. D., Hampton, J. R., & Mitchell, J. R. A. (1978). A randomized trial of home-versus-hospital management for patients with suspected myocardial infarction. *The Lancet*, *1*(8069), 837–841.

Hill, J. D., Hampton, J. R., & Mitchell, J. R. A. (1979). Home or hospital for myocardial infarction—Who cares? *American Heart Journal*, *98*, 545–547.

Hopper, S. V., Miller, J. P., Birge, C., & Swift, J. (1984). A randomized study of the impact of home health aides on diabetic control and utilization patterns. *American Journal of Public Health*, *74*, 600–602.

Hu, T., Huang, L., & Cartwright, W. S. (1986). Evaluation of the costs of caring for the senile demented elderly: A pilot study. *The Gerontologist*, *26*, 158–163.

Hughes, S. L. (1985). Apples and oranges? A review of evaluations of community-based long-term care. *Health Services Research*, *20*, 461–488.

Hughes, S. L., Cordray, D. S., & Spiker, V. A. (1984). Evaluation of a long-term home care program. *Medical Care*, *22*, 460–475.

Hughes, S. L., Manheim, L. M., Edelman, P. L., & Conrad, K. J. (1987). Impact of long-term home care on hospital and nursing home use and cost. *Health Services Research*, *22*, 19–47.

Iams, J. D., Johnson, F. F., O'Shaughnessy, R. W., & West, L. C. (1987). A prospective random trial of home uterine activity monitoring in pregnancies at increased risk of preterm labor. *American Journal of Obstetrics and Gynecology*, *157*, 638–643.

James, M. L., Hudson, C. N., Gebski, V. J., Browne, L. H., Andrews, G. R., Crisp, S. E., Palmer, D., & Beresford, J. L. (1987). An evaluation of planned early postnatal transfer home with nursing support. *Medical Journal of Australia*, *147*, 434–438.

King, F. E., Figge, J., & Harman, P. (1986). The elderly coping at home: A study of continuity of nursing care. *Journal of Advanced Nursing*, *11*, 41–46.

Kornblatt, E. S., Fisher, M. E., & MacMillen, D. J. (1985). Impact of DRGs on home health nursing. *Quality Review Board*, *7*, 290–294.

Kramer, A. M., Shaughnessy, P. W., & Pettigrew, M. L. (1985). Cost-effectiveness implications based on a comparison of nursing home and home health case mix. *Health Services Research*, *20*, 387–405.

Kun, S., & Warburton, D. (1987). Telephone assessment of parents' knowledge of home-care treatments and readmission outcomes for high-risk infants and toddlers. *American Journal of Diseases in Children*, *141*, 888–892.

Legh-Smith, J., Wade, D. T., & Langton-Hewer, R. (1986). Services for stroke patients one year after stroke. *Journal of Epidemiology and Community Health*, *40*, 161–165.

Liang, M. H., Partridge, A. J., Larson, M. G., Gall, V., Taylor, J., Berkman, C., Master, R., Feltin, M., & Taylor, J. (1984). Evaluation of comprehensive rehabilitation services for elderly homebound patients with arthritis and orthopedic disability. *Arthritis and Rheumatism*, *27*, 258–266.

Make, B.J., & Gilmartin, M. E. (1986). Rehabilitation and home care for ventilator-assisted individuals. *Clinics in Chest Medicine*, *7*, 679–691.

Marshall, J. (1987). A review of the discharge preparation and initial community support given to families of neonates after surgical intensive care. *Intensive Care Nursing, 2*(3), 101–106.

Martin, K. (1988). Research in home care. *Nursing Clinics of North America, 23*, 373–385.

Martinson, I. M., Moldow, D. G., Armstrong, G. D., Henry, W. F., Nesbit, M. E., & Kersey, J. H. (1986). Home care for children dying of cancer. *Research in Nursing & Health, 9*, 11–16.

McClelland, E., & Kelly, K. (1980). Characteristics of clients referred for post-hospital health care. *Home Health Review, 3*(3), 11–22.

McCusker, J., & Stoddard, A. M. (1987). Effects of an expanding home care program for the terminally ill. *Medical Care, 25*, 373–385.

Medical Research Council Working Party. (1981). Long term domiciliary oxygen therapy with chronic hypoxic cor pulmonale complicating chronic bronchitis and emphysema. *The Lancet, 1*(8222), 681–685.

Moore, J. E., Eisenberg, M. S., Andresen, E., Cummins, R. O., Hallstrom, A., & Litwin, P. (1986). Home placement of automatic external defibrillators among survivors of ventricular fibrillation. *Annals of Emergency Medicine, 15*, 811–812.

Mundinger, M. O. (1983). *Home care controversy: Too little, too late, too costly.* Rockville, MD: Aspen.

Nieweg, R., Greidanus, J., & de Vries, E. G. E. (1987). A patient education program for a continuous infusion regimen on an outpatient basis. *Cancer Nursing, 10*, 177–182.

Olds, D. L., Henderson, C. R., Tatelbaum, R., & Chamberlin, R. (1988). Improving the life-course development of socially disadvantaged mothers: A randomized trial of nurse home visitation. *American Journal of Public Health, 78*, 1436–1445.

Pai, S., & Nagarajaiah. (1982). Treatment of schizophrenic patients in their homes through a visiting nurse—Some issues in the nurse's training. *International Journal of Nursing Studies, 19*(3), 167–172.

Pasquale, D. K. (1987). A basis for prospective payment for home care. *Image: Journal of Nursing Scholarship, 19*, 186–191.

Pasquale, D. K. (1988). Characteristics of Medicare-eligible home care clients. *Public Health Nursing, 5*, 129–134.

Paykel, E. S., Mangen, S. P., Griffith, J. H., & Burns, T. P. (1982). Community psychiatric nursing for neurotic patients: A controlled trial. *British Journal of Psychiatry, 140*, 573–581.

Peters, D. A. (1988). Development of a Community Health Intensity Rating Scale. *Nursing Research, 37*, 202–207.

Pringle, D., & Taylor, D. (1984). Palliative care in the home: Does it work? *Canadian Nurse, 80*(6), 26–29.

Schulze, M. W., & Koerner, B. L. (1987). Attitudes of community health nurses toward maternal and child health nursing: Development of an instrument. *Journal of Professional Nursing, 3*, 347–353.

Sebern, M. D. (1986). Pressure ulcer management in home health care: Efficacy and cost effectiveness of moisture vapor permeable dressing. *Archives of Physical Medicine and Rehabilitation, 67*, 726–729.

Soldo, B. J. (1985). In-home services for the dependent elderly. *Research on Aging, 7*, 281–304.

Spiegel, A. D. (1987). *Home health care* (2nd ed.). Owings Mills, MD: Rynd.

Stanek, L. M. (1987). An analysis of professional nurse burnout in two selected nursing care settings. *Journal of Nursing Administration, 17*(5), 3, 29.

Stiller, S. B. (1988). Success and difficulty in high-tech home care. *Public Health Nursing, 5,* 68–75.

Stiver, H. G., Trosky, S. K., Cote, D. D., & Oruck, J. L. (1982). Self-administration of intravenous antibiotics: An efficient, cost-effective home care program. *Canadian Medical Association Journal, 127,* 207–211.

Stone, R. (1986). Aging in the eighties, age 65 years and over—Use of community services. *NCHS Advance Data, 124,* 1–7 [DHHS Publication No. (PHS) 86–1250].

Storfjell, J. (1987). *A quantification model for home health care nursing visits.* Unpublished doctoral dissertation, The University of Michigan, Ann Arbor.

U.S. Department of Health and Human Services. (1988). *Sixth report to the President and Congress on the status of health personnel in the United States* (DHHS Publication No. HRS-P-OD-88-1). Washington, DC: Author.

U.S. General Accounting Office. (1979). *Home health care services—Tighter controls needed* (Report # GAO/HRD-81-155). Washington, DC: Author.

Vinciguerra, V., Degnan, T. J., Budman, D. R., Brody, R. S., Moore, T., Sciortino, A., & O'Connell, M. (1986). Comparative cost analysis of home and hospital treatment. *Progress in Clinical and Biological Research, 216,* 155–164.

Vinciguerra, V., Degnan, T. J., Sciortino, A., O'Connell, M., Moore, T., Brody, R., Budman, D., Eng, M., & Carlton, D. (1986). A comparative assessment of home versus hospital comprehensive treatment for advanced cancer patients. *Journal of Clinical Oncology, 4,* 1521–1528.

von Windeguth, B., Urbano, M. T., Hayes, J. S., & Martyn, K. K. (1988). Analysis of infant risk factors documented by public health nurses. *Public Health Nursing, 5,* 165–169.

Wade, D. T., Langton-Hewer, R., Skilbeck, C. E., Bainton, D., & Burns-Cox, C. (1985). Controlled trial of a home-care service for acute stroke patients. *The Lancet, 1*(8424), 323–326.

Young, K. M., & Fisher, C. R. (1980). Medicare episodes of illness: A study of hospital, skilled nursing facility, and home health agency care. *Health Care Financing Review, 2*(2), 1–23.

Zimmer, J. G., Groth-Juncker, A., & McCusker, J. (1985). A randomized controlled study of a home health care team. *American Journal of Public Health, 75,* 134–141.

Chapter 6

Nursing Administration Research, Part One: Pluralities of Persons

PHYLLIS R. SCHULTZ
SCHOOL OF NURSING
UNIVERSITY OF WASHINGTON

KAREN L. MILLER
THE CHILDREN'S HOSPITAL AND
SCHOOL OF NURSING
UNIVERSITY OF COLORADO HEALTH SCIENCES CENTER

CONTENTS

Nursing administration research has been slow to develop, partly due to confusion within the nursing community about the focus of nursing administration relative to other specialty domains. Support of clinical practice and research was thought to be the primary role of the nurse

We acknowledge the assistance of Patricia Budd, Andrea Lacina, Donna Koch, and Lee Richards for their help with assessing the reliability in selection of the articles.

133

administrator, with little emphasis on the unique practice and research in the domain of nursing administration (DeGroot, Ferketich, & Larson, 1987). In addition, the narrow definition of nursing practice as limited to the clinical has contributed to profound deficits in theory and knowledge development in nursing administration practice (Jennings & Meleis, 1988).

Since the advent of major economic and regulatory changes in the health care industry, there has been increased acceptance of nursing administration as a practice of nursing that is crucial to the survival of the nursing profession. Recognition of the value of administration within nursing has led nurse scholars to identify the need for specific research and theory development in this specialty domain (Henry, 1989; Henry et al., 1987; Jennings & Meleis, 1988). This chapter is an integrative review of the research-based nursing literature conducted as a beginning effort to explicate theory from existing nursing administration research.

DEFINITION OF CLIENT IN NURSING ADMINISTRATION

The review was guided by a definition of *client* in nursing administration practice as "more than one" and twofold: (a) pluralities of persons associated with nursing care delivery systems regardless of setting, and (b) nursing care delivery systems as organizations, that is, as social interactional units (Schultz, 1987). This definition gives rise to a framework that includes four components pertaining to pluralities of persons associated with a nursing organization: persons served, professional staff or persons who provide the nursing care, support staff or persons who support the direct care providers, and administrative staff or persons who direct, facilitate, and coordinate delivery of nursing services. The focus of this chapter is on nursing research about pluralities of persons associated with nursing organizations.

The framework also includes five components pertaining to the organization as an interactional unit: resource management, costs of delivering care, quality of care and nursing processes, subcomponent interaction, and social and technical work environment. A chapter to follow in Volume 9 will be focused on components of the nursing organization as an interactional unit.

Key concepts and generalizations identified from the abstracted studies are used to outline a foundation for nursing administration.

They are congruent with assumptions and defining concepts of *person, environment, health,* and *nursing* (Meleis, 1985).

RETRIEVAL, SELECTION, AND REVIEW PROCESS

Given the scope of reported research in the nursing literature, the major criterion for selection of an article was whether the title reflected the subject matter of one of the nine components of the definitional framework described above. These components are conceptually consistent with the recently established definition of nursing administration research:

> Nursing administration research is the scientific inquiry of factors that affect the effective and efficient organization and delivery of high-quality nursing services. This research is concerned with the systematic examination of the relationship between nursing services and patient care and with assessment of the elements of nursing care delivery systems. (American Organization of Nurse Executives, 1987, p. 1)

The search was limited to studies in which at least one of the investigators was a nurse researcher. Research articles germane to the nine components that appeared in earlier volumes of the *Annual Review of Nursing Research* were excluded, for example, nursing staff turnover, socialization and roles in nursing, assessment of quality of nursing care, leadership, costs of nursing care, and nursing diagnosis.

Nursing administration as a specialty was given renewed emphasis in the profession in the mid-1970s (Blair, 1976). This history provided the rationale for limiting the review to the decade from 1977 to 1987. Calls for increased attention to research in nursing administration were also present in the literature at that time (Dimond & Slothower, 1978; Jacox, 1978). Manual reviews were conducted of the following nursing journals: *Image* (1977 to 1987), *Journal of Community Health Nursing* (1984 to 1987), *Journal of Nursing Administration* (1977 to 1987), *Nursing Administration Quarterly* (1977 to 1987), *Nursing Economics* (1983 to 1987), *Nursing & Health Care, Nursing Management* (1981 to 1987), *Nursing Outlook* (1977 to 1987), *Nursing Research* (1977 to 1987), *Public Health Nursing* (1984 to 1987), *Research in Nursing & Health* (1978 to 1987) and *Western Journal of Nursing Research* (1979 to 1987). Initial selection resulted in 536 articles. Of these, only four articles pertained to support personnel associated with nursing care organizations, and no articles were located that were focused on interactions among the subunits of nursing care organizations or interactions between the nursing division and other units of the health care organization. Thus this chapter and the chapter to come in Volume 9 include eight of the original nine nursing administration framework components (Schultz, 1987).

Of the 525 articles, 230 were focused on topics covered in previously published or scheduled chapters in the *Annual Review of Nursing Research*. These were omitted, leaving 102 for this chapter (Part I), a review of research on pluralities of persons, and 193 for the chapter in a later volume (Part II), a review of research on the nursing care organization. Interrater reliability by the average congruency percentage method (Waltz, Strickland, & Lenz, 1984) was accomplished for selection of articles with the aid of four graduate students in nursing. Categorizing was conducted independently by the two authors.

Each article was abstracted according to identical topics: purpose, topic, code words, framework, design, sample, tools, metrics, data collection, procedures, results, discussion, implications, and comments. For comments, the authors judged the overall quality of the research and evaluated the likelihood that the study could be replicated on the basis of the report. The abstracts were entered into a flat text data base to facilitate analysis.

PLURALITIES OF PERSONS

For nursing administration research to generate knowledge congruent with nursing as a discipline, the focus of study must have involved some dimension of one or more of the four defining concepts and have been consistent with the discipline's values and assumptions. The term *plurality of persons* was identified from conceptual analysis to extend the meaning of the concept of *client* in nursing to include persons in the plural as well as to retain the orientation of human beings in the fullest sense of their personhood and agency (Schultz, 1987). Who are the pluralities of persons appropriate for study in nursing administration research? To be more than a mere aggregate of individual humans, the persons of interest must be associated with a nursing care organization in some way, that is, affiliated with the organization, and must define themselves in part by that affiliation (Schultz, 1987).

Persons Served

Of the 102 articles pertaining to pluralities of persons associated with nursing care organizations, 30 studies were focused on persons served. As clients of nursing care organizations, they included several types such as the terminally ill or handicapped (Byrne, 1984; Dixon, 1981; Reed, 1987), those at risk for falls (Walshe & Rosen, 1979), or those with medical problems, for example, cancer, cardiac, or psychiatric diagnoses (Byrne & Edeani, 1984; Molde & Baker, 1985; Topf, Dambacher, & Roper, 1979). Nurse investigators also studied persons served according to several demographic characteristics such as ethnic groups or minorities (Flaskerud, 1984), and age groups, such as preschool (Pidgeon, 1981), school-age (Riffee, 1981; Savedra & Tesler, 1981), adolescents (Craft, 1981), and the elderly (Chang, 1978; Fife, Solomon, & Stanton, 1984; Foreman, 1987; Janken, Reynolds, & Swiech, 1986; Kim, 1986; Mion, Frengley, & Adams, 1986; Ryden, 1984; Swarzbeck, 1983; Williams et al., 1985). Other ways of categorizing clients were according to association with a specific type of nursing organization or setting for care, for example, hospital (Geden & Begeman, 1981; Nojima et al., 1987), emergency department (Lauck & Bigelow, 1983), general medical–surgical unit (Brown, Buchanan, & Hsu, 1978; Volicer & Burns, 1977) or nursing clinic (Muhlenkamp, Brown, & Sands, 1985); or those with needs at discharge or for home care (Ballard & McNamara, 1983; Garrard, Dowd, Dorsey, & Shapiro, 1987; Kromminga & Ostwald, 1987). A number of these pluralities were vulnerable populations, such as the very young, the very old, those from diverse cultures, and those whose access to health services is limited. Those specific groups have been recommended for research in nursing administration (Henry et al., 1987, p. 313).

The purpose of eight articles was to report factors predictive of need for nursing care or types of nursing interventions such as living arrangements and personal care support; learning needs; nutritional, mobility, or elimination needs; spiritual support; threats to self-esteem; and stress and mental confusion (Ballard & McNamara, 1983; Byrne, 1984; Kim, 1986; Mion, Frengley, & Adams, 1986; Reed, 1987;

Riffee, 1981; Volicer & Burns, 1977; Williams et al., 1985). Eight were on various health behaviors such as seeking illness prevention or health promotion (Muhlenkamp et al., 1985), enactment of the sick role (Brown et al., 1978), identification with handicapped persons (Dixon, 1981), or follow-through from the emergency department (Lauck & Bigelow, 1983). In three studies differences in perceptions or attitudes between client groups and nursing personnel were examined (Byrne & Edeani, 1984; Flaskerud, 1984; Topf, Dambacher, & Roper, 1979). Three articles were reports of tool development or testing, for example, comparing the reliability and validity of three mental status tools (Foreman, 1987), developing and testing a checklist for discharge planning (Kromminga & Ostwald, 1987) and post-hospital care (Garrard et al., 1987). One group of investigators tested nursing theory on perceptions of time and space in hospitalized volunteers (Nojima et al., 1987). All these studies represent efforts on the part of nurse researchers to identify systematically the types of care needed by various groups or pluralities of persons and factors predicting nursing care needs.

Health conditions prescriptive for nursing care reflected in these studies include confusion and general mental status, falls, life stress, hospital stress, style of coping, health beliefs and behaviors, functional problems, medications, general morale, dependency, self-esteem status, general well-being, perceptions and preferences regarding care, and presenting complaints. Systematic appraisal of these conditions through research was oriented toward identifying predictors, criteria, trends, length of stay, cultural elements, and patterns of coordination of nursing care.

The primary characteristic of these studies has been a focus on commonalities of problems across groups of persons rather than individual problems and responses. Several generalizations pertaining to clients as pluralities of persons can serve as a beginning knowledge base of this type of plurality. Level and type of health status are predictive of number and type of nursing visits and patterns of care (Ballard & McNamara, 1983; Muhlenkamp et al., 1985). Persons in need of hospice and home care can be identified prior to discharge from acute-care hospitals (Ballard & McNamara, 1983; Garrard et al., 1987; Kromminga & Ostwald, 1987). The hospitalized injured and ill elderly who are mildly or severely confused, who have diuretics prescribed, and who attempt to get out of bed to use the bathroom are at greatest risk for falls and for injuries due to falls. The health risk to these persons can be reduced through specific staffing patterns and staff orientation (Fife et al., 1984; Janken et al., 1986; Swarzbeck, 1983; Walshe & Rosen, 1979). In general, factors influencing care strategies and nursing interventions of clients include age; type of pathophysiology including medical diagnoses; knowledge of illness and treatment; level of education; self-control; self-esteem; personal preferences for time, space, and interpersonal interaction; and mental status.

Several qualities of these studies are indicators of a generally firm base on which to plan nursing care modalities and delivery strategies and to design further research. The investigators have provided a knowledge that is primarily descriptive of various populations' demographic or medical characteristics or need for nursing care. Some type of theoretical framework was identifiable in 20 of the 30 studies. In 10, a survey design was used (Ballard & McNamara, 1983; Byrne, 1984; Craft, 1981; Geden & Begeman, 1981; Kromminga & Ostwald, 1987; Lauck & Bigelow, 1983; Molde & Baker, 1985; Pidgeon, 1981; Ryden, 1984; Walshe & Rosen, 1979). Two studies were exploratory in nature (Craft, 1981; Savedra & Tesler, 1981), and in seven the researchers used descriptive designs (Byrne & Edeani, 1984; Kromminga & Ostwald, 1987; Mion et al., 1986; Pidgeon, 1981; Swarzbeck, 1983; Volicer & Burns, 1977; Walshe & Rosen, 1979). Five investigators included correlational analyses to strengthen the design (Ballard & McNamara, 1983; Chang, 1978; Muhlenkamp et al., 1985; Ryden, 1984; Volicer & Burns, 1977); five studies used comparison groups (Brown et al., 1978; Dixon, 1981; Flaskerud, 1984; Janken et al., 1986; Nojima et al., 1987; Reed, 1987; Riffee, 1981; Topf et al., 1979; Williams et al., 1985); one used a quasi-experimental approach (Kim, 1986); and one designed an experimental study (Fife et al., 1984). In five, hypotheses were tested (Flaskerud, 1984; Kim, 1986; Nojima et al., 1987; Riffee, 1981; Topf et al., 1979). In several studies more than one design was used. Seven authors reported random selection of subjects, 13 used some form of systematic selection that was not random, and 10 reported convenience samples. In 21 studies, correlations, multiple regression, or analysis of variance (ANOVA) were used to analyze the data; chi square and t-test were used in 5; descriptive statistics were reported in 8; and 1 researcher used qualitative analyses. In those studies in which instrument development or instrument comparisons were the focus, the researchers used reliability and validity estimation procedures with appropriate statistics.

The weakest quality of the studies was a lack of reliability or validity estimates for the tools reported. This lack, combined with nonrandom convenience samples, contributed to a judgment that 12 could not be replicated on the basis of the report. Eighteen were judged as adequate for replication, especially if the survey questionnaire or other instruments had been tested for reliability and validity and the estimates were available in the report.

Unfortunately, only a few investigators studied the amount and type or pattern of nursing services in relation to health outcomes of particular types of persons served. This focus is a priority for future research (American Organization of Nurse Executives, 1987; Henry et al., 1987).

Professional Personnel

Thirty-nine articles pertaining to professional personnel associated with nursing care organizations met the criteria for selection. All were reports of research in which registered nurses were the subjects except one. In the latter study, licensed practical nurses were included with registered nurses who had various types of educational backgrounds such as associate, baccalaureate, or master's degrees. Twenty of the 39 studies were focused on aspects of professional nurses as employees or members of a work force. Topics included labor force participation and employment patterns (Greenleaf, 1983; Knopf, 1983; Nolan, 1985); recruitment, incentives, and factors of discontent (Beyers, Mullner, Byre, & Whitehead, 1983a; Deets & Froebe, 1984; Ginzberg, Patray, Ostow, & Brann, 1982; Munro, 1983; Weisman, Dear, Alexander, & Chase, 1981); career preferences and success (Hefferin & Kleinknecht, 1986; Zimmerman & Yeaworth, 1986); orientation to position and to changes due to displacement or relocation (Barnes, Harmon, & Kish, 1986; Beyers et al., 1983a; Ireson & Powers, 1987); clinical levels and roles including physician-hired nurses (Beyers, Mullner, Byre, & Whitehead, 1983b, Felder & Riesch, 1980; Rustia, Wilson & Quinn, 1985); salaries (Beyers et al., 1983b; Spitzer & Bolton, 1984); absenteeism (Curran & Curran, 1987; D. S. Miller & Norton, 1986); and use of orientation of supplemental nurses (Boyer, 1979; Prescott, 1986). A second topic addressed by researchers of 10 studies pertained to various types of physical and psychological health problems including health defined eudaimonistically (Smith, 1981) as the need for intellectual and creative growth (Harrison,

1987). Personal, lifestyle, and work-related characteristics of nurses with back injuries were studied by Owen and Damron (1984). Conditions of a psychological or mental health nature included burnout and stress (Cronin-Stubbs & Schaffner, 1985; Rich & Rich, 1987), addiction to smoking and drugs (Feldman & Richard, 1986; Hutchinson, 1987; Wagner, 1985), depression (van Servellen, Soccorso, Palermo, & Faude, 1985), and verbal abuse suffered on the job (Cox, 1987).

Seven studies were focused on various aspects of nursing practice as perceived by professional nurses, such as behaviors that can be identified as uniquely nursing (Bradley, 1983), knowledge-informed practice (Clark & Lenberg, 1980), clinical decision making (Prescott, Dennis, & Jacox, 1987), confidence in the care of ethnically diverse groups (Bernal & Froman, 1987), measurement and evaluation of job performance (Koerner, 1981; Stull, 1986), and ability of nurses to be person-centered in their care (K. A. Wallston, Cohen, B. S. Wallston, Smith, & Devellis, 1978). The least number of studies were directed toward describing the extent to which nurses joined or participated in professional associations, political activities, or collective bargaining (Beletz, 1982; Moore & Oakley, 1983; Yeager & Kline, 1983).

The topics of these studies provide some of the content areas of knowledge required in the practice of nursing administration—the qualities of the largest group of staff in a nursing organization. For example, the findings from these studies (1977 to 1987) provide clues for explaining the repeated cycles of shortage that have characterized nursing. Unlike women in other predominantly female occupations, nurses tend to leave the work force after their children are raised (Greenleaf, 1983); 25% stop work after 15 years (Knopf, 1983). Their work life patterns are complex, including a stable pattern of continuous employment and career advancement, a double-track pattern of work and family, and an interrupted pattern of work/raise family/ return to work (Nolan, 1985). Aspects of the work environment such as job stress and burnout seem to be associated with various types of health problems among nurses such as smoking, chemical dependency, and physical problems such as back injuries (Cronin-Stubbs & Schaffner, 1985; Feldman & Richard, 1986; Hutchinson, 1987; Owen & Damron, 1984; Rich & Rich, 1987). In the mid-1980s Deets and Froebe (1984) identified professional recognition, autonomy, working conditions, and compensation as accounting for nearly 40% of the variance of factors contributing to nurses entering and staying in the work force.

What is known about nurses, how is it known, how warrantable is it (Schultz & Meleis, 1988)? The studies provided primarily descriptive information as summarized above. Quantitative survey design was used in 20 of the 39 studies. Other designs included grounded theory (Hutchinson, 1987), qualitative exploratory (Nolan, 1985; Weisman et al., 1981), qualitative survey (Boyer, 1979; Clark & Lenberg, 1980; Prescott et al., 1987), comparison groups with quantitative measures (Barnes et al., 1986), longitudinal cohort (Knopf, 1983), ex post facto with existing data (Greenleaf, 1983; Munro, 1983), correlational (Cronin-Stubbs & Schaffner, 1985; Deets & Froebe, 1984; Moore & Oakley, 1983), and experimental (Curran & Curran, 1987; Stull, 1986). In two articles the authors reported instrument development (Bradley, 1983; Hefferin & Kleinknecht, 1986), and two investigators incorporated hypotheses-testing with other designs (Koerner, 1981; Wallston et al., 1978).

No theoretical framework was reported in 21 studies, and many investigators cited only previous research related to the topic. One researcher used the grounded theory research approach and generated a theory to explain chemical dependency among nurses (Hutchinson, 1987). Of those investigators reporting the use of a theoretical framework, none were based on a nursing theory or conceptual framework. Theories from management (Barnes et al., 1986; Curran & Curran, 1987; Ireson & Powers, 1987), occupational psychology (Bernal & Froman, 1987; Cronin-Stubbs & Schaffner, 1985; Rich & Rich, 1987; Stull, 1986), sociology of the professions (Harrison, 1987; Prescott et al., 1987; Weisman et al., 1981), and complex organizations (Clark & Lenberg, 1980; Deets & Froebe, 1984; Greenleaf, 1983; Koerner, 1981; Yeager & Kline, 1983) were more frequently represented. One study was based on Kramer's (1974) research on "reality shock" (Hefferin & Kleinknecht, 1986), which meant the study was built on previous nursing research but not a nursing framework.

Random samples of respondents were used in 12 studies, a block quota sampling frame in one study, and convenience, purpose, or other nonrandom samples in 26 studies. Instruments were designed by the investigators or identified from the research literature. Reliability or validity properties of instruments from previous research were reported in six studies: internal consistency for scales used in the studies in six, test–retest or split-half reliability in two, interrater estimates in two, and content validity in one. Twenty-two of the 39 reports contained no information about reliability or validity of the instrumentation.

In the largest number of studies ($n = 22$), descriptive statistics were used to summarize the results. Some type of qualitative analysis was used in four studies. The t test for group comparisons was reported in two studies, and three investigators used correlations. In nine studies multiple regression, ANOVA, or factor analysis was used.

Eleven of the 39 studies (28%) were judged by the reviewers to be especially difficult to replicate, primarily because of problems with methodology such as the ones summarized above. Nine others could be replicated.

Support Personnel

Review of 12 nursing journals yielded only four reports of research focused on support personnel associated with nursing organizations. Support personnel as a category of pluralities of persons included those who worked in job classifications that supported the core mission of the nursing organization, that is, nursing care. Such job classifications would include secretaries, administrative assistants, ward clerks, nurses' aides and assistants, orderlies, and persons who maintain the physical plant of the nursing department or agency.

Of the four retrieved articles, one was focused on nurse aides and assistants in a hospital setting (Brief, Aldag, & Jacox, 1978); two were about psychiatric nursing assistants (Depp, Arnold, Dawkins, & Selzer, 1983; Floyd, 1983), and one pertained to job performance of a nursing home staff consisting primarily of licensed practical nurses and nurse assistants (Sheridan, Fairchild, & Kaas, 1983). Three of the 4 studies were quantitative surveys, and the other was a report of instrument development using the multitrait/multimethod strategy. Two of the 3 surveys contained descriptions of task characteristics, intrinsic factors, extrinsic factors, and institutional factors related to job satisfaction in hospital nursing assistants (Brief et al., 1978) or psychiatric nursing assistants (Floyd, 1983). In the third survey the investigators identified personal–attitudinal and ward-related organizational factors predictive of 6- and 12-month job tenure of psychiatric nursing assistants (Depp et al., 1983). The researchers who reported the instrument development study attempted to design behavior-anchored scales for rating nursing job performance among nursing home staff (Sheridan et al., 1983).

Findings from these studies provided clues to important job-related characteristics of support personnel associated with nursing care organizations. Hospital nurse assistant task characteristics in the early part of the decade included maintaining general personal hygiene, meeting patient-specific needs, and admitting patients. Nurse assistant tasks also included selected nonroutine types of activities such as gastrostomy feedings, colostomy dressings, patient care planning, and maintaining intake and output recordings (Brief et al., 1978). Personal attitude and training variables were significant determinants of psychiatric assistants' tenure in the first few months of employment, whereas ward and organizational factors gained importance at 12 months (Depp et al., 1983). Intrinsic factors such as good working relationships, importance of helping others, and contributing to patient recovery and extrinsic factors such as periodic pay increases, amount of compensation including retirement, and scheduling contributed to job satisfaction among psychiatric nursing aides (Floyd, 1983). In the same study the quality of the medical staff and availability of equipment and personnel were cited as institutional factors.

It was judged that three of the four studies could be replicated on the basis of the report, although two of the three survey reports contained no tool reliability or validity estimates. One investigator mentioned pilot studies, but no reliability or validity estimates were included in the report. All four studies were based on theoretical formulations from the management and occupational psychology literature rather than nursing. None of the samples were random. The fit of the research questions with the design and statistics contributed to the warrantability of the knowledge generated in these studies.

Administrative Personnel

Eighteen of the 29 articles pertaining to administrative personnel were focused on the chief nurse executive of various health care delivery systems (Archer, 1983; Claus & Binger, 1978; Farley, 1987; Feldman & Daly-Gawenda, 1985; Freund, 1985b; Friss, 1983; Harrison & Roth, 1987; Henry & Moody, 1986; Hillestad, 1984; Johnson, 1987; Porter, 1987; Poulin, 1984; Price, Simms, & Pfoutz, 1987; Reynolds, 1987; Sargis, 1978; Schofield, 1986; Sietsma & Spradley, 1987; Simms, Price, & Pfoutz, 1985). One of the striking aspects of this group was the variety of names and titles used to denote the highest level of nurse in the organization. The titles included director of nursing, vice-president for nursing, chief nurse executive, nurse service director, nurse administrator, and nursing leader. Other persons included in studies of administrative personnel were assistant or associate directors of nursing (Archer & Goehner, 1981; Brenner et al., 1986; Duffy & Gold, 1980; Fine, 1983; Price, 1984; Price et al., 1987; Simms et al., 1985), supervisors (Buccheri, 1986; Greaves & Loquist, 1983), and head nurses (Beaman, 1986; Stahl, Querin, Rudy, & Crawford, 1983). Delineation of roles and titles among these groups was not always clear, and the evidence suggested the potential for role conflict and differences in expectations in the practice situation (Stahl et al., 1983).

Significant for this group of studies was the clear specification of the type of organization with which the administrative personnel were associated. Almost all ($n = 25$) the studies were specified according to type of hospital or health care delivery system. The most frequently specified work environment and context for these studies was the acute-care hospital (Beaman, 1986; Johnson, 1987; Price et al., 1987; Reynolds, 1987; Sargis, 1978; Schofield, 1986; Simms et al., 1985; Simms, Pfoutz, & Price, 1986; Stahl et al., 1983), although various types and sizes of hospitals were used including psychiatric, government, and university-affiliated hospitals. Other health care delivery systems identified were rural hospitals, long-term care facilities, home care systems, and city and county health departments.

In general, the research interest was about the social and demographic characteristics of administrative personnel, with several authors citing the lack of adequate demographic knowledge about nurses working as administrators. For this reason most of these studies included the collection of demographic data as a priority, particularly the earlier research of this group (1978–1981). However, only Claus and Binger (1978) stated the purpose of the study to be the collection of demographic data. Poulin (1984) described the profile of the nurse executive in the mid-1980s as a single woman between 50 and 59 years of age, graduate of a diploma program, in present position 5 years, career-oriented, and with a corporate title. This profile reflected changes since the early 1970s commensurate with responsibility, increased power, more budget control, control over nonnursing departments, decentralization, and the pressures of legal constraints and regulations.

Despite the fact that most studies were focused on the chief nurse executive as subject, research interests and issues varied. Topics included the concepts of power and communication (Farley, 1987), decision making (Harrison & Roth, 1987), turnover and tenure (Freund, 1985b), situational assessment techniques (Porter, 1987), orientation process (Schofield, 1986), politics (Archer, 1983; Archer

& Goehner, 1981), ethics (Sietsma & Spradley, 1987), caring (Brenner et al., 1986), organizational commitment (Friss, 1983), professional loneliness (Hillestad, 1984), collective bargaining (Sargis, 1978), and social and demographic characteristics (Claus & Binger, 1978). The greatest concentration of studies on one topic was related to the role, behaviors, and functions of administrators in director of nursing positions (Feldman & Daly-Gawenda, 1985; Henry & Moody, 1986; Poulin, 1984; Price et al., 1987; Simms et al., 1985, 1986) or head nurse positions (Beaman, 1986; Buccheri, 1986; Stahl et al., 1983). Delineation of administrative functions and behaviors was directed generally toward identifying nonclinical nursing roles and specifying appropriate educational preparation for nurses in administration (Johnson, 1987; Simms et al., 1985). The second most frequent topic of interest in the studies of admininstrative personnel was education, with recommendations for graduate curricula in nursing administration (Duffy & Gold, 1980; Fine, 1983; Freund, 1985a; Greaves & Loquist, 1983; Johnson, 1987; Price, 1984; Reynolds, 1987).

Taken as a whole, these studies provide evidence that nursing administration is a highly dynamic activity with increasing scope and complexity involving leadership, management of human and capital resources, dynamic interaction with members of the entire health care organization, and ethical decision making, an activity requiring many competencies (Price, 1984). The nurse administrator's role is a lonely one due in part to the focus on promoting high-quality patient care as contrasted with the institutional survival focus of other administrators (Hillestad, 1984). Educational preparation is required in the content areas of management theory and principles, organizational theory and politics, fiscal and budgetary management, marketing and planning, performance appraisal and other personnel matters, nursing theory and advances in clinical care, health policy, legal and regulatory issues and constraints, and ethics (Duffy & Gold, 1980; Greaves & Loquist, 1983; Johnson, 1987; Porter, 1987; Reynolds, 1987; Sietsma & Bradley, 1987). Skills in political strategies (Archer, 1983; Archer & Goehner, 1981) and empowering nursing staff (Harrison & Roth, 1987) are considered critical. The 43% turnover rate reported by Freund (1985b) suggests that nurse administrators are at high risk for stress and conflict, particularly in eras of retrenchment like those of the early 1980s (Feldman & Daly-Gawenda, 1985). The high turnover rate also may be due to the lack of career planning (Price et al., 1987). Knowledge of changing demographics in populations (Simms et al., 1986) and technical changes in clinical nursing such as the demand for long-term care is more important than maintaining clinical competencies per se (Price, 1984). Henry and Moody (1986) documented the extent to which decision making by nurse administrators in small rural hospitals can be based on more detailed information and direct observations than those in large urban hospitals. Networking (Hillestad, 1984) and mentoring are important for combating isolation and fostering effectiveness, especially because of the fact that many nurse administrators acquire their expertise from job experience (Price et al., 1987; Reynolds, 1987). Nurse administrators are more satisfied with their jobs than middle managers or staff nurses (Buccheri, 1986) and are in high demand (Fine, 1983).

The credibility of these studies of administrative personnel rests on the explication of the nature of the nursing administrator's role and nursing administration practice as outlined above. In seven of the studies investigators reported conceptual frameworks that related to the topic of interest. The majority of studies ($n = 24$) indicated some review of related literature without reference to a specific conceptual framework. No investigator used or evolved nursing theory per se, and in five articles the authors did not cite related literature or a conceptual basis for the research from any source. One investigator stated that the purpose of the investigation was to generate theory. The report contained a description of diagnostic reasoning in nursing administration practice in order to develop theory related to population group administrative diagnosis (Porter, 1987). This effort is in keeping with current attempts by nurse administrators and educators to develop nursing theory specific to the domain of nursing administration (Jennings & Meleis, 1988; Meleis & Jennings, 1989; Miller, 1988). There were two reports of a study designed from a grounded theory approach, but the investigators did not include theory in the report (Simms et al., 1985, 1986).

The plurality of administrative personnel was examined primarily through descriptive survey design (Archer, 1983; Archer & Goehner, 1981; Beaman, 1986; Buccheri, 1986; Claus & Binger, 1978; Duffy & Gold, 1980; Farley, 1987; Freund, 1985a, 1985b; Friss, 1983; Greaves & Loquist, 1983; Harrison & Roth, 1987; Henry & Moody, 1986; Hillestad, 1984; Johnson, 1987; Price, 1984; Reynolds, 1987; Sargis, 1978; Schofield, 1986; Sietsma & Spradley, 1987; Stahl et al., 1983) and 19 authors or teams summarized and reported the data with descriptive statistics. Most researchers utilized questionnaire format. Several investigators used qualitative approaches such as grounded theory (Porter, 1987; Price et al., 1987; Simms et al., 1985, 1986), structured interview

(Feldman & Daly-Gawenda, 1985; Poulin, 1984), and ethnography (Brenner et al., 1986) and reported the findings in terms of categories and themes. One study on the impact of continuing education was designed as evalution research incorporating pre- and posttesting and t-test comparisons (Greaves & Loquist, 1983). This was the only article in which the researchers specifically addressed measurement of outcomes, an important indicator of quality and effectiveness of the nurse administrator's role in current health care delivery systems. Chi-square (Beaman, 1986; Johnson, 1987; Sargis, 1978), Pearson correlations (Buccheri, 1986; Farley, 1987; Hillestad, 1984; Stahl et al., 1983), and ANOVA (Buccheri, 1986; Harrison & Roth, 1987; Hillestad, 1984; Price, 1984) also were used appropriately for research questions and designs.

Samples included both random ($n = 12$) and convenience ($n = 7$). Ten researchers used a qualitative design approach. In general, the samples in about half of the studies of this plurality were not delineated adequately, and nearly all the tools were not tested for reliability and validity prior to use. Face validity procedures and piloting of tools were mentioned in some articles, but specific reliability and validity estimates were not provided. These deficits in the reports make replication difficult.

Nineteen (65.5%) of the total number of studies focused on administrative personnel were judged difficult, if not impossible, to replicate, largely because of the lack of information on the instruments used for data collection. Because 10 of these studies were qualitative in design, auditability and credibility would be the important considerations (Sandelowski, 1986). Despite weaknesses in methodology in many of the studies, the research provided valuable information on administrative personnel in nursing and some insight into the nature of their practice. The potential for research-based theory development is reflected in these research reports even though variables in nursing administration research are difficult to specify and to measure (Dimond & Slothower, 1978; Jacox, 1978).

THEORY DEVELOPMENT

The studies in this review provide an important research base on which to generate theory about the pluralities of persons associated with nursing care organizations (Schultz, 1987). Relationships can be inferred among nursing's defining concepts such as persons with health, persons with environment, persons with nursing therapeutics, person–environment–health, and person–environment–health–nursing (Fawcett, 1984). For example, investigators of professional nurses have related their personal characteristics with their health-threatening behaviors or conditions such as smoking, depression, drug dependency, stress, and back injuries (Cronin-Stubbs & Schaffner, 1985; Feldman & Richard, 1986; Hutchinson, 1987; Owen & Damron, 1984; van Servellen et al., 1985). In some studies the findings linked the environment, specifically the work environment, to these health-threatening behaviors and conditions as well (Cronin-Stubbs & Schaffner, 1985; van Servellen et al., 1985). In nearly all the studies pertaining to administrative personnel the person is related with the environment vis-à-vis his/her work role. Other person–environment studies included the exploration of the importance of personal space preferences among hospitalized adults (Geden & Begeman, 1981), professional nurses' responses to relocation (Ireson & Power, 1987), and the Koerner (1981) study of the relationship between job performance and organizational environment.

Health behaviors were associated with number and type of nursing visits (Muhlenkamp et al., 1985), a finding that demonstrates the relationship between the concepts of person and nursing. The study by Fife et al. (1984) on falls in hospitalized elderly and nursing strategies designed to prevent them illustrates a relationship among the concepts of person, environment, nursing, and health, with health defined clinically as the prevention of injury (Smith, 1981).

In these studies the researchers provide the empirical evidence from which a contribution to nursing theory can be elucidated; heretofore such studies have been "conceptualized as management research not grounded in nursing theory" (Schultz, 1987, p. 82). When the meaning of *client* is extended beyond individual persons to include pluralities of persons associated with nursing organizations, nursing theory and knowledge development can be advanced in new ways. For example, the studies provided evidence for understanding the commonalities of health behaviors and conditions across groups, such as stress, dependency, and needs for growth (Harrison, 1987); this evidence may suggest to the reader the fallacy of viewing "persons served" as patients who are "sick" cared for by nurses who are "well." Another example is that knowledge about group identification, such as defining oneself as "handicapped," has implications for the formulation and functioning of support groups (Dixon, 1981). This phenomenon may be extended to other groups with specific health problems, including support groups for hospitalized patients with particular diagnoses or groups of professional nurses such as those with drug dependencies or burnout. Specifically, members of support groups need to identify with the group to realize the therapeutic potential of the group (Sampson & Marthas, 1977). In addition, generating theory from a profile of persons served can provide a knowledge base for designing preventive nursing care strategies for particular groups of patients, such as the elderly at risk for falls (Fife et al., 1984; Swarzbeck, 1983; Walshe & Rosen, 1979). The profile of nurse administrators as a group (Poulin, 1984) can lead to organizational theories about isolation and turnover, which in turn can be the basis for administrative policy formulation and evaluation.

If nursing is to be recognized as a discipline, nursing theory cannot be restricted to explanations of the interactions of individual clients with individual nurse providers. Rather, the defining concepts of the discipline and the profession's values and orientation must direct attention to the phenomena of interest congruent with nursing's domain (Schultz & Meleis, 1988). When understood from this perspective, theory about the various pluralities of persons associated with nursing care organizations can contribute to nursing's knowledge base.

RESEARCH ISSUES AND FUTURE DIRECTIONS

Seventy-five percent of the articles retrieved for this review were published from 1983 through 1987, indicating a substantial increase in research in this domain in the second half of the decade. Twenty-seven percent were published in the *Journal of Nursing Administration* and 24% in *Nursing Research*. Sixty-three percent of the articles pertaining to persons served (19) appeared in the literature from 1983 through 1987 and 40% were located in *Nursing Research*. Of the research reports on professional personnel, 77% were published in the second half of the decade, with 31% retrieved from the *Journal of Nursing Administration* and another 28% from *Nursing Research*. Three of the four articles in which support personnel were the subjects were published in the last five years of the decade. Over half (52%) of the articles pertaining to administrative personnel were published in the *Journal of Nursing Administration*, and 86% were retrieved from the 1983 through 1987 literature.

Although the facts cited above suggest a substantial increase in research on topics of importance to nursing administration theory and knowledge development, several directions can be charted for future research. First, substantial innovation in research approaches is needed to illuminate the dimensions of nursing administration practice in nursing and in health care delivery. Traditional quantitative surveys have described clearly the increasingly heavy demands, responsibilities, and complexities, but the full meaning of the practice and its congruence with nursing's domain concepts and assumptions remain unexplored. Second, in regard to what is known about professional nurses affiliated with nursing care organizations, there is a great disparity between the evidence from cited research and the degree to which the evidence has failed to impact organizational policy and administrative decision making. The evidence clearly directs administrative policy formulation away from traditional hierarchical structure and patriarchal management styles and toward decentralized, professional models in which nursing's knowledge-based practice and contributions to healing and health are recognized. Future research must be focused on this disparity. Investigators need to discover the demographic, economic, organizational, and professional forces preventing the recruitment and retention of persons into the profession. Third, there is substantial need for continued research focused on the health characteristics of persons served by nursing care organizations and the commonalities of their needs for nursing care. These studies should be guided by current nursing theories, assumptions, and values in order to extend nursing's contribution to the health of populations beyond the traditional treatment of clinical problems and toward the enhancement of eudaimonistic health. Such studies also will require innovation in research approaches, design, and measurement in order to generate credible knowledge on which to base nursing care modalities and new delivery strategies. Fourth, the lack of research focused on the characteristics and growth needs of nonprofessional support personnel associated with nursing care organizations must be corrected. Nurse administrators can make human resource decisions based on the research of others. But the discipline's orientation to holism and respect for person demand study by nurse investigators of these personnel so that nurse managers can have the knowledge to help support personnel realize their potential with nursing's goals, values, and practice. The studies that were found clearly indicate that nurse's aides and assistants do see themselves as contributing to patient care and take satisfaction and motivation from these task identities. Nurse administrators need more of this kind of information so that they can create work environments that sustain support personnel in these kinds of interests and commitments.

Perhaps the most telling discovery from this integrative review is the frequent lack of theoretical frameworks within which to ask the research questions, frameworks that are congruent with nursing's defining concepts and domain assumptions. There is need for inquiries that are addressed to the defining concepts individually and in combination and are reflective of the patterns of knowledge that characterize nursing as a discipline (Schultz & Meleis, 1988). In addition to well-designed empirical studies that can be replicated for understanding the nurse administrator's complex practice, inquiries should include conceptual analysis of such concepts as power and administrative caring. Explicating the currently implicit theoretical dimensions of nursing administrative decision making and political processes would contribute to more effective practice and education. Studies are needed of the ethical dimensions of administrative practice. Research on the esthetic needs of persons served that enhance their recoveries and sustain their health would advance the knowledge base consistent with nursing's patterns of knowing (Schultz & Meleis, 1988). The personal, ethical, and esthetic needs of persons served and of professional, support, and administrative personnel are open topics for fruitful inquiry.

REFERENCES

American Organization of Nurse Executives. (1987). *National nursing administration priorities study.* Chicago, IL: American Hospital Association.

Archer, S. E. (1983). A study of nurse administrators' political participation. *Western Journal of Nursing Research, 5,* 65–75.

Archer, S. E., & Goehner, P. A. (1981). Acquiring political clout: Guidelines for nurse administrators. *Journal of Nursing Administration, 11*(12), 49–55.

Ballard, S., & McNamara, R. (1983). Quantifying nursing needs in home health care. *Nursing Research, 32,* 236–241.

Barnes, D. J., Harmon, P., & Kish, J. P. (1986). A displacement orientation program—Effects on transferred nurses. *Journal of Nursing Administration, 16*(7, 8), 45–50.

Beaman, A. L. (1986). What do first-line nursing managers do? *Journal of Nursing Administration, 16*(5), 6–9.

Beletz, E. E. (1982). Nurses participation in bargaining units. *Nursing Management, 13*(10), 48–58.

Bernal, H., & Froman, R. (1987). The confidence of community health nurses in caring for ethnically diverse population. *Image: Journal of Nursing Scholarship, 19*, 201–203.

Beyers, M., Mullner, R., Byre, C. S., & Whitehead, S. F. (1983a). Results of the nursing personnel survey, Part 1: RN recruitment and orientation. *Journal of Nursing Administration, 13*(4), 34–37.

Beyers, M., Mullner, R., Byre, C. S., & Whitehead, S. F. (1983b). Results of the nursing personnel survey, Part 2: RN vacancies and turnover. *Journal of Nursing Administration, 13*(5), 26–31.

Blair, E. M. (1976). Needed: Nursing administration leaders. *Nursing Outlook, 24*, 550–554.

Boyer, C. M. (1979). The use of supplemental nurses: Why, where, how? *Journal of Nursing Administration, 9*(3), 56–60.

Bradley, J. C. (1983). Nurses' attitudes dimensions of nursing practice. *Nursing Research, 32*, 110–114.

Brenner, P., Boyd, C., Thompson, T. C., Marz, M. S., Buerhouse, P., & Leininger, M. (1986). The care symposium—Considerations for nursing administrators. *Journal of Nursing Administration, 16*(1), 25–30.

Brief, A. P., Aldag, R. J., & Jacox, A. (1978). A study: The impact of task characteristics on employee response in hospital nursing. *Nursing Administration Quarterly, 2*(4), 107–114.

Brown, J. S., Buchanan, D., & Hsu, L. N. (1978). Sex differences in sick role behavior during hospitalization after open heart surgery. *Research in Nursing & Health, 1*, 37–48.

Buccheri, R. C. (1986). Nursing supervision: A new look at an old role. *Nursing Administration Quarterly, 11*(1), 11–25.

Byrne, C. M. (1984). An assessment of the need for hospice services in a rural area. *Journal of Community Health Nursing, 1*(1), 59–64.

Byrne, T. J., & Edeani, D. (1984). Knowledge of medical terminology among hospital patients. *Nursing Research, 33*, 178–181.

Chang, B. L. (1978). Generalized expectancy, situational perception and morale among institutionalized aged. *Nursing Research, 27*, 316–323.

Clark, N. M., & Lenberg, C. B. (1980). Knowledge-informed behavior and the nursing culture: A preliminary study. *Nursing Research, 29*, 244–249.

Claus, K. E., & Binger, J. E. (1978). How directors of nursing service use and share the nursing literature. *Journal of Nursing Administration, 8*(11), 17–21.

Cox, H. C. (1987). Verbal abuse in nursing: Report of a study. *Nursing Management, 18*(11), 47–50.

Craft, M. (1981). Preferences of hospitalized adolescents for information providers. *Nursing Research, 30*, 205–211.

Cronin-Stubbs, D., & Schaffner, J. W. (1985). Professional impairment: Strategies for managing the troubled nurse. *Nursing Administration Quarterly, 9*(3), 44–54.

Curran, M. A., & Curran, K. E. (1987). Gambling away absenteeism. *Journal of Nursing Administration, 17*(12), 28–31.

Deets, C., & Froebe, D. J. (1984). Incentives for nurse employment. *Nursing Research, 33,* 242–246.

DeGroot, H. A., Ferketich, S. L., & Larson, P. J. (1987). Theory development in a non-university service setting. *Journal of Nursing Administration, 17*(4), 38–44.

Depp, F. C., Arnold, E., Dawkins, J., & Selzer, N. (1983). Predicting tenure decision of psychiatric nursing assistants: Individual and work-related factors. *Research in Nursing & Health, 6,* 53–59.

Dimond, M., & Slothower, L. (1978). Research in nursing administration: A neglected issue. *Nursing Administration Quarterly, 2*(4), 1–8.

Dixon, J. K. (1981). Group-self identification and physical handicap: Implication for patient support groups. *Research in Nursing & Health, 4,* 299–308.

Duffy, M. E., & Gold, N. E. (1980). Education for nursing administration: What investment yields highest returns? *Journal of Nursing Administration, 10*(9), 31–38.

Farley, M. (1987). Power orientations and communication style of managers and nonmanagers. *Research in Nursing & Health, 10,* 197–202.

Fawcett, J. (1984). Hallmarks of success in nursing research. *Advances in Nursing Science, 7*(3), 1–11.

Felder, E., & Riesch, S. (1980). The status of minority nurses in Wisconsin. *Nursing Research, 29,* 60–61.

Feldman, B. M., & Richard, E. (1986). Prevalence of nurse smokers and variables identified with successful and unsuccessful smoking cessation. *Research in Nursing & Health, 9,* 131–138.

Feldman, J., & Daly-Gawenda, D. (1985). Retrenchment—How nurse executives cope. *Journal of Nursing Administration, 15*(6), 31–37.

Fife, D. D., Solomon, P., & Stanton, M. (1984). A risk/falls program: Code orange for success. *Nursing Management, 15*(11), 50–53.

Fine, R. B. (1983). The supply and demand of nursing administrators. *Nursing & Health Care, 4,* 10–15.

Flaskerud, J. H. (1984). A comparison of perceptions of problematic behavior by six minority groups and mental health professionals. *Nursing Research, 33,* 190–197.

Floyd, G. J. (1983). Psychiatric nursing aides: A job satisfaction profile. *Nursing Management, 14*(9), 36–40.

Foreman, M. D. (1987). Reliability and validity of mental status questionnaires in elderly hospitalized patients. *Nursing Research, 36,* 216–220.

Freund, C. M. (1985a). Director of nursing effectiveness—DON and CEO perspectives and implications for education. *Journal of Nursing Administration, 15*(6), 25–30.

Freund, C. M. (1985b). The tenure of directors of nursing. *Journal of Nursing Administration, 15*(2), 11–15.

Friss, L. (1983). Organization commitment and job involvement of directors of nursing services. *Nursing Administration Quarterly, 7*(2), 1–10.

Garrard, J., Dowd, B. E., Dorsey, B., & Shapiro, J. (1987). A checklist to assess the need for home health care: Instrument development and validation. *Public Health Nursing, 4,* 212–218.

Geden, E. A., & Begeman, A. V. (1981). Personal space preferences of hospitalized adults. *Research in Nursing & Health, 4,* 237–241.

Ginzberg, E., Patray, J., Ostow, M., & Brann, E. A. (1982). Nurse discontent: The search for realistic solutions. *Journal of Nursing Administration, 12*(11), 7–11.

Greaves, P. E., & Loquist, R. S. (1983). Impact evaluation: A competency-based approach. *Nursing Administration Quarterly, 7*(3), 81–86.

Greenleaf, N. P. (1983). Labor force participation among registered nurses and women in comparable occupations. *Nursing Research, 32,* 306–311.

Harrison, J. K. (1987). Tuning in to the growth needs of registered nurses. *Nursing Economics, 5,* 297–303.

Harrison, J. K., & Roth, P. A. (1987). Empowering nursing in multihospital systems. *Nursing Economics, 5,* 70–76.

Hefferin, E. A., & Kleinknecht, M. K. (1986). Development of the Nursing Career Preference Inventory. *Nursing Research, 35,* 44–48.

Henry, B. M. (1989). Research themes and methods for nursing administration. In B. Henry, C. Arndt, M. DiVincenti, & A. Marriner-Tomey (Eds.), *Dimensions and issues in nursing administration* (pp. 247–250). Boston, MA: Blackwell Scientific Publications.

Henry, B. M., & Moody, L. E. (1986). Nursing administration to small rural hospitals. *Journal of Nursing Administration, 16*(7, 8), 37–44.

Henry, B. M., Moody, E., Pendergast, J., O'Donnell, J., Hutchinson, S., & Scully, G. (1987). Delineating nursing administration research priorities using three futures methods. *Nursing Research, 36,* 309–314.

Jacox, A. (1978). Where are the researchers in nursing administration? *Nursing Administration Quarterly, 2*(4), 54–56.

Janken, J. K., Reynolds, B. A., & Swiech, K. (1986). Patient falls in the acute care setting: Identifying risk factors. *Nursing Research, 35,* 215–219.

Jennings, B. M., & Meleis, A. I. (1988). Nursing theory and administrative practice: Agenda for the 1990's. *Advances in Nursing Science, 10*(3), 56–69.

Johnson, M. S. (1987). Preparing nurse executives for financial management. *Nursing Administration Quarterly, 12*(1), 67–73.

Kim, K. K. (1986). Response time and health care learning of elderly patients. *Research in Nursing & Health, 9,* 233–239.

Knopf, L. (1983). Registered nurses fifteen years after graduations: Findings from the nurse career-pattern study. *Nursing & Health Care, 4,* 72–76.

Koerner, B. L. (1981). Selected correlates of job performance of community health nurses. *Nursing Research, 30,* 43–48.

Kramer, M. (1974). *Reality shock: Why nurses leave nursing.* St. Louis, MO: Mosby.

Kromminga, S. K., & Ostwald, S. K. (1987). The public health nurse as a discharge planner: Patients' perceptions of the discharge process. *Public Health Nursing, 4,* 224–229.

Lauck, B. W., & Bigelow, D. A. (1983). Why patients follow through on referrals from the emergency room and why they don't. *Nursing Research, 32,* 186–187.

Meleis, A. I. (1985). *Theoretical nursing: Development and progress.* Philadelphia, PA: J. B. Lippincott.

Meleis, A. I., & Jennings, B. M. (1989). Theoretical nursing administration:

Today's challenges, tomorrow's bridges. In B. Henry, C. Arndt, C. M. DiVincenti, & A. Marriner (Eds.), *Dimensions and issues in nursing administration* (pp. 7–18). Boston, MA: Blackwell Scientific Publications.

Miller, D. S., & Norton, V. M. (1986). Absenteeism—Nursing service's albatross. *Journal of Nursing Administration, 16*(3), 38–42.

Miller, K. L. (1988). *Feminist ideology in nursing: A foundational inquiry.* Unpublished doctoral dissertation, University of Colorado, Boulder.

Mion, L., Frengley, J. D., & Adams, M. (1986). Nursing patients 75 years and older. *Nursing Management, 17*(9), 24–28.

Molde, S., & Baker, D. (1985). Explaining primary care visits. *Image: The Journal of Nursing Scholarship, 17,* 72–76.

Moore, E., & Oakley, D. (1983). Nurses, political participation and attitudes toward reforms in the health care system. *Nursing & Health Care, 4,* 504–507.

Muhlenkamp, A. F., Brown, N. J., & Sands, D. (1985). Determinants of health promotion activities in nursing clinic clients. *Nursing Research, 34,* 327–332.

Munro, B. H. (1983). Young graduate nurses: Who are they and what do they want? *Journal of Nursing Administration, 13*(6), 21–26.

Nojima, Y., Oda, A., Nishii, H., Fukui, J., Seo, K., & Akiyoshi, H. (1987). Perception of time among Japanese inpatients. *Western Journal of Nursing Research, 9,* 288–300.

Nolan, J. W. (1985). Work patterns of midlife female nurses. *Nursing Research, 34,* 150–154.

Owen, B. D., & Damron, C. F. (1984). Personal characteristics and back injury among hospital nursing personnel. *Research in Nursing & Health, 7,* 305–313.

Pidgeon, V. (1981). Functions of preschool children's questions in coping with hospitalizations. *Research in Nursing & Health, 4,* 229–235.

Porter, E. J. (1987). Administrative diagnosis—Implications for the public's health. *Public Health Nursing, 4,* 247–256.

Poulin, M. A. (1984). The nurse executive role—A structural and functional analysis. *Journal of Nursing Administration, 14*(2), 9–14.

Prescott, P. A. (1986). Use of nurses from supplemental services: Implications for hospitals. *Nursing Administration Quarterly, 11*(1), 81–88.

Prescott, P. A., Dennis, K. E., & Jacox, A. K. (1987). Clinical decision making of staff nurses. *Image: Journal of Nursing Scholarship, 19,* 56–62.

Price, S. A. (1984). Master's programs preparing nursing administrators—What are the essential components? *Journal of Nursing Administration, 14*(1), 11–17.

Price, S. A., Simms, L. M., & Pfoutz, S. K. (1987). Career advancement of nurse executives: Planned or accidental? *Nursing Outlook, 35,* 236–238.

Reed, P. G. (1987). Spirituality and well-being in terminally ill hospitalized adults. *Research in Nursing & Health, 10,* 335–344.

Reynolds, B. J. (1987). Directors of nursing service: How well prepared are they? *Nursing Outlook, 35,* 274–287.

Rich, V. L., & Rich, A. R. (1987). Personality hardiness and burnout in female staff nurses. *Image: Journal of Nursing Scholarship, 19,* 63–66.

Riffee, D. M. (1981). Self-esteem changes in hospitalized school-age children. *Nursing Research, 30,* 94–97.

Rustia, J., Wilson, C., & Quinn, J. (1985). Use of physician-hired nurses. *Journal of Nursing Administration, 15*(9), 35–40.

Ryden, M. B. (1984). Morale and perceived control in institutionalized elderly. *Nursing Research, 33,* 130–136.

Sampson, E. E., & Marthas, M. S. (1977). *Group process for the health professions.* New York: Wiley.

Sandelowski, M. (1986). The problem of rigor in qualitative research. *Advances in Nursing Science, 3*(3), 27–37.

Sargis, N. M. (1978). Will nursing directors' attitudes affect future collective bargaining? *Journal of Nursing Administration, 8*(12), 21–26.

Savedra, M., & Tesler, M. (1981). Coping strategies of hopsitalized school-age children. *Western Journal of Nursing Research, 3,* 371–384.

Schofield, V. M. (1986). Orientation of nurse executives. *Journal of Nursing Administration, 16*(11), 13–17.

Schultz, P. R. (1987). When client means more than one: Extending the foundational concept of person. *Advances in Nursing Sciences, 10*(1), 71–86.

Schultz, P. R., & Meleis, A. I. (1988). Nursing epistemology: Traditions, insights, questions. *Image: Journal of Nursing Scholarship, 20,* 217–221.

Sheridan, J. E., Fairchild, T. J., & Kaas, M. (1983). Assessing the job performance of nursing home staff. *Nursing Research, 32,* 102–107.

Sietsma, M. R., & Spradley, B. W. (1987). Ethics and administrative decision making. *Journal of Nursing Administration, 17*(4), 28–32.

Simms, L. M., Pfoutz, S. K., & Price, S. C. (1986). Caring for older people: A challenge for nurse administrators. *Nursing Outlook, 34,* 145–148.

Simms, L. M., Price, S. A., & Pfoutz, S. K. (1985). Nurse executives: Functions and priorities. *Nursing Economics, 3,* 238–244.

Smith, J. B. (1981). The idea of health: A philosophical inquiry. *Advances in Nursing Science, 3*(3), 43–50.

Spitzer, R. B., & Boston, L. B. (1984). Attitudes toward equitable pay. *Nursing Management, 15*(6), 32–38.

Stahl, L. D., Querin, J. J., Rudy, E. B., & Crawford, M. A. (1983). Head nurses' activities and supervisors' expectations: The research. *Journal of Nursing Administration, 13*(6), 27–33.

Stull, M. K. (1986). Staff nurse performance—Effects of goal-setting and performance feedback. *Journal of Nursing Administration, 16*(7, 8), 26–30.

Swarzbeck, E. M. (1983). The problems of falls in the elderly. *Nursing Management, 14*(12), 34–38.

Topf, M., Dambacher, B., & Roper, J. (1979). Quality of interpersonal style among hospitalized psychiatric patients. *Western Journal of Nursing Research, 1,* 163–178.

van Servellen, G. M., Soccorso, E. A., Palermo, K., & Faude, K. (1985). Depression in hospital nurses: Implications for nurse managers. *Nursing Administration Quarterly, 9*(3), 74–84.

Volicer, B. J., & Burns, M. W. (1977). Preexisting correlates of hospital stress. *Nursing Research, 26,* 408–415.

Wagner, T. J. (1985). Smoking behavior of nurses in Western New York. *Nursing Research, 34,* 58–60.

Wallston, K. A., Cohen, B. D., Wallston, B. S., Smith, R. A., & Devellis, B. M. (1978). Increasing nurses' person-centeredness. *Nursing Research, 27,* 156–159.

Walshe, A., & Rosen, H. (1979). A study of patient falls from bed. *Journal of Nursing Administration, 3*(5), 31–35.

Waltz, C. F., Strickland, O. L., & Lenz, E. R. (1984). *Measurement in nursing research.* Philadelphia: F. A. Davis.

Weisman, C. S., Dear, M. R., Alexander, C. S., & Chase, G. A. (1981). Employment patterns among newly hired hospital staff nurses: Comparison of nursing graduates and experienced nurses. *Nursing Research, 30,* 188–191.

Williams, M. A., Campbell, E. B., Raynor, W. J., Musholt, M. A., Mlynarczyk, S. M., & Crane, L. F. (1985). Predictors of acute confusional states in hospitalized elderly patients. *Research in Nursing & Health, 8,* 31–40.

Yeager, S. J., & Kline, M. (1983). Professional association membership of nurses: Factors affecting membership and the decision to join an association. *Research in Nursing & Health, 6,* 45–52.

Zimmerman, L., & Yeaworth, R. (1986). Factors influencing career success in nursing. *Research in Nursing & Health, 9,* 179–185.

PART III

Research on
Nursing Education

Chapter 7

Education for Critical Care Nursing

MARGUERITE R. KINNEY
SCHOOL OF NURSING
UNIVERSITY OF ALABAMA AT BIRMINGHAM

CONTENTS

Conceptual Model
AACN Educational Standards Task Force
Questions for the Review
Assessment of Educational Needs
Planning for Critical Care Nursing Education
Implementation of the Educational Process
Evaluation of the Educational Process
Factors Influencing Critical Care Nursing Education
Conclusions
Recommendations for Future Research

Though Florence Nightingale recognized the need to place the sickest soldiers closest to the nurse, it was not until the end of World War II that critical care units began to be integrated into the structure of America's general hospitals. In the 1960s, coronary care experiments in Kansas City (Day, 1963) and in Philadelphia (Meltzer, 1965) demonstrated that the specialized knowledge and skill of nurses could result in decreased mortality rates for patients hospitalized with acute myocardial infarction. As the demand for nurses with specialized knowledge and skills increased, educational offerings flourished, and presently attention is being given to the process and structure of critical care nursing education.

The purpose of this review was to examine the reported research related to critical care nursing education in order to evaluate the extent to which the educational process in this specialty of nursing practice is grounded in research. The review was limited to research conducted and reported in the United States over a 17-year period from 1971 to 1988. No research reports were found in the published literature prior to 1971. Three major sources served to direct the review: MEDLINE, *Dissertation Abstracts International*, and *Education Standards for Critical Care Nursing* (Alspach et al., 1986). In addition, the reference citations for all literature reviewed were examined. A total of 72 titles were identified and examined, revealing 14 research reports that comprised this review.

CONCEPTUAL MODEL

The American Association of Critical Care Nurses' (AACN) Conceptual Model for the Education Standards for Critical Care Nursing served as a framework for the review (Figure 7-1). The conceptual model was derived from the explicit underlying assumptions and operational definitions incorporated into the model. In the model, the term *education* refers to education that occurs after entry into professional nursing practice, and basic preparation in nursing is assumed. Critical care nursing is defined as the specialty within nursing that deals specifically with human responses to life-threatening problems (AACN, 1984).

The conceptual model is comprised of two major elements: the *sphere* of critical care nursing resting on a *base* of general education principles. The construct of general education includes learning theories and principles of adult education; a basic assumption is that the responsibility for learning rests with the learner. The sphere encompassing critical care nursing practice includes competent practice and the educational process leading to competent practice. The goal of quality care for critically ill patients is common to critical care nursing and critical care nursing education. Further structure for the model is provided by the *Standards for Nursing Care of the Critically Ill* (Thierer et al., 1981), the AACN Scope of Practice Statement (Disch, 1980), AACN's Principles of Practice (Bertram, 1982), and the nursing process. Effective use of the nursing process is based on an assumption that a knowledge base and psychomotor skills have

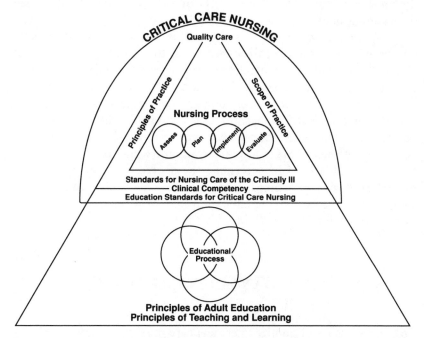

Figure 7-1. Conceptual model for the Education Standards for Critical Care Nursing.

Source: Kuhn, R. C., Canobbio, M. M., Alspach, J. G., Roberts, W. L. & Turzan, L. (1985). Education standards for critical care nursing-conceptual framework. *Heart & Lung, 14*(2), 188. Reprinted with permission of C. V. Mosby Co.

been acquired. The requisite knowledge and skills for critical care nursing practice are provided in *Core Curriculum for Critical Care Nursing* (Alspach & Williams, 1985).

Education provides the process by which competency is attained and maintained. Critical care education is provided both within and outside the critical care environment and is defined as "education directed at facilitating application of the knowledge, skills, and attitudes required for competent critical care nursing practice" (Alspach, 1983). The educational process incorporates assessment, planning, implementation, and evaluation, thereby influencing critical care nursing practice and culminating in the delivery of high-quality patient care. Because the components of the educational process are dynamic and interacting, the model depicts the components in an overlapping manner.

Educational assessment is defined as an organized, systematic determination of the educational needs of the critical care nurse and includes collection, organization, analysis, and validation of data related to educational needs. Data are obtained from a variety of sources, such as the learner or the employer. *Planning* encompasses prioritizing the identified learning needs and delineating instructional objectives to guide the educational endeavor. *Implementation* is the execution of the educational plan. *Evaluation* may be summative or formative and is used to determine the degree to which the desired outcomes have been realized. Finally, factors that influence the provision of critical care nursing education may be categorized as institutional, professional, or individual.

AACN EDUCATION STANDARDS TASK FORCE

To address issues of quality in critical care nursing education, AACN established the Education Standards Task Force in 1981 that was charged with developing education standards for critical care nursing. The Task Force conducted an extensive review of the literature and published a characterization of the state of critical care nursing education (Roberts et al., 1986).

Critical care nursing education was described as being provided in three distinct settings: academic, service, and private. In the academic setting, critical care nursing education is offered in basic or graduate nursing curricula or in the form of continuing education. In the service setting, critical care nursing education is offered as staff development that includes orientation, in-service education, and continuing education. In the private setting, critical care nursing education is provided in the form of continuing education by professional associations and societies and by commercial organizations.

The report of the Task Force characterized critical care nursing education in the three settings according to the following features: (a) rationale for providing critical care nursing education; (b) providers of critical care nursing education; (c) methods of providing critical care nursing education; (d) expected outcomes; (e) evaluation methods; (f) institutional, individual, and professional factors impinging on critical care nursing education; and (g) existing standards that affect critical care nursing education.

Great variability and inconsistency were found in the process and structure of critical care nursing education across the three settings. Although the rationale was consistent across settings, that is, to prepare competent critical care practitioners, specific short-term and intermediate goals were not shared, nor were universal standards and guidelines adopted. No consensus was found related to qualifications of educators, methods of facilitating learning, or core knowledge or skills requisite for competent practice. No data could be found relating positive patient outcomes to competency in nursing practice; thus the influence of education on critical care nursing practice was judged largely unknown or inferred. Evaluation of critical care nursing education varied considerably. A lack of published information was found, including descriptions of valid and reliable instruments for evaluation. A number of institutional, professional, and individual factors were described as affecting the provision of critical care nursing education, but the full impact of the factors could not be discerned. Finally, although no standards were found to address critical care nursing education in the private setting, criteria for appraisal of academic nursing programs and for service settings were found to have implications for critical care nursing education.

The Task Force acknowledged the need for standards for critical care nursing education, and these were developed and published in 1986 (Alspach et al., 1986). Further, the Task Force identified a number of broad research questions designed to answer questions related to competencies, educational and evaluative methods, structural components, outcomes, assessment, and influencing factors. The questions were:

1. What minimal competencies (cognitive, psychomotor, or affective) are necessary to ensure safe and effective clinical practice for critical care nurses? What competencies define the boundaries of intermediate or advanced practice of critical care nursing? What competencies define specialization in critical care nursing?

2. To what degree and in what form are the various educational methods, formats, and vehicles effective in facilitating attainment of desired critical care competencies?

3. What evaluative methods and instruments will provide valid and reliable measures of competency in critical care nursing?

4. What structural components are required to effect a valid critical care educational process? More specifically, what is optimal with regard to the following factors: (a) qualifications, requirements, and responsibilities of institutional and individual providers of critical care education in each educational setting; (b) educational resources (material, financial, and human) required for critical care education; (c) environmental and instructional supports; (d) staffing and instructor/learner ratios; and (e) organizational and managerial support for critical care education?

5. What patient outcomes correlate positively with competency in critical care nursing?

6. Which methods of assessment will ensure valid, accurate, and reliable identification of learning needs of critical care nurses?

7. To what extent and in what manner do various institutional, professional, and individual factors influence the provision of critical care nursing education?

QUESTIONS FOR THE REVIEW

Inasmuch as the educational process incorporates the major elements of assessment, planning, implementation, and evaluation, these four sequential elements will serve to organize the questions addressed in this review.

1. What is the state of the art of educational assessment in critical care nursing?
    a. What learning needs have been identified?
    b. What methods have been employed to assess learning needs?
    c. What instruments are available to assist with assessing learning needs?
2. How have the identified learning needs been prioritized?
3. What expected outcomes have been described?
4. What is the state of the art in implementation of the educational plan?
    a. What execution strategies have been described?

5. To what degree have the desired outcomes of critical care nursing education been realized?
6. What institutional, professional, and individual factors have been identified and demonstrated to influence the provision of critical care nursing education?

ASSESSMENT OF EDUCATIONAL NEEDS

Torrez (1972) conducted the earliest study related to assessment of educational needs, specifically educational needs of coronary care nurses. In this descriptive study, Torrez asked the following questions: (a) Are planned coronary care education programs necessary for nurses? (b) Which nurses are willing to participate in such programs? (c) Is there a difference in the needs and desires regarding planned teaching programs of nurses in teaching and nonteaching hospitals or of nurses who received planned preparation prior to employment and those who did not? (d) How will recommendations for a coronary care program made by nurses with previous preparation compare with recommendations of nurses with no previous preparation?

The sample consisted of 60 registered nurses employed in four general hospitals in the Southwest. A questionnaire was developed and distributed, with 40 subjects responding (66.6%). Generalizability of the findings is limited by the small, nonrepresentative sample as well as by the questionable psychometric properties of the instrument and the nonsystematic error introduced in the method employed for data collection. Analysis of the data was not addressed to differences among nurses differing in experience or in employment setting, but a list of topics recommended for inclusion in a teaching program was generated.

Canfield (1981, 1982) employed a descriptive design for the following purposes: (a) to identify the clinical competencies necessary for beginning-level critical care nurses; (b) to determine the relationship between baccalaureate educators' and nursing service employers' perceptions of clinical competencies necessary for beginning-level critical care nurses; (c) to determine the relationship between clinical content taught in baccalaureate programs and in in-service programs for the preparation of beginning critical care nurses; (d) to examine the assignment of newly graduated baccalaureate nurses to critical care settings; (e) to examine what, if any, education or experience were required for assignment to a critical care unit; and (f) to identify what, if any, problems educators encountered in providing clinical experience for students in critical care settings. The sample consisted of 57 nurse educators and 107 nursing employers from one Western state. Clinical competencies were derived from a list of 21 theoretical content areas endorsed by AACN as appropriate for nursing students in critical care. A panel of experts defined specific competencies for each of the 21 content areas, yielding a list of 102 clinical competencies.

Canfield (1981, 1982) found significant differences between educators and employers in perceptions of competencies necessary for beginning critical care nurses. A significant difference also was found between clinical content taught in the two settings. New graduates were hired for beginning positions in critical care by 40% of employers, and 68.5% of employers judged new graduates as having been prepared unsatisfactorily for employment in critical care. Major difficulties in assigning students to critical care were not reported. The major findings of this study were the lack of agreement about which competencies are necessary for beginning practice in critical care and the inevitable dissatisfaction of employers with the preparation of newly graduated nurses for practice in this setting.

The generalizability of the findings again is limited by the nonrepresentative sample and the psychometric properties of the instrument. As in the Torrez (1972) study, a list of topics about which a critical care nurse should be knowledgeable and a list of desirable skills were generated.

In an effort to assess new graduates' perceptions of their ability to work in a critical care setting, a random sample of 100 graduates from baccalaureate degree, associate degree, and diploma programs in nursing who had applied to take the state board examination in one state were mailed a self-report questionnaire (Jackle, Ceronsky, & Petersen, 1977; Petersen, Jackle, & Ceronsky, 1977). Eighty-nine subjects responded (89%). Face validity of the questionnaire was judged by a panel of experts. Subjects were asked to provide information about their educational program and their preparation for critical care nursing practice. A list of topics was presented, and subjects were asked to indicate the extent to which they had theoretical instruction and practice. Findings revealed a number of topics in which the subjects reported little or no instruction and practice.

Though content and face validity of the instrument were judged, there is no indication that the instrument was reliable. Further, the limited responses available to respondents made interpretation of the findings difficult.

Only one instrument for assessing knowledge in critical care nursing was identified (Toth, 1984; Toth & Ritchey, 1982). The Basic Knowledge Assessment Tool (BKAT) is a 90-item multiple choice and fill-in-the-blank test that yields seven subscales: (a) cardiovascular, (b) monitoring lines, (c) pulmonary, (d) neurology, (e) endocrine, (f) renal, and (g) nutrition combined with miscellaneous content. Content for the test was identified from a review of the literature, interviews with critical care nurses, and suggestions from physicians and experts in critical care nursing practice and education. Questions were designed to test recall and application of basic information, with a total score of 90 points possible. Validity was estimated by a panel of experts, and factor analysis was used for validation of the subscale items. Reliability was estimated using Cronbach's alpha (.86 for the total test; .81 for the cardiovascular subscale; and .71 for the noncardiovascular scales). The test has been found to discriminate between newly graduated nurses and nurses with experience. The BKAT has been revised and presently consists of 100 items with seven subscales. The modified version (BKAT-2) has been demonstrated to be a valid and reliable instrument for assessing knowledge basic to safe practice in critical care nursing (Toth, 1984).

In summary, very few studies have been done to identify the educational needs of critical care nurses. Though lists of needs have been generated from self-report instruments, literature review, and an expert panel, there is little empirical evidence to support these lists. One instrument is available to test basic knowledge in critical care nursing.

PLANNING FOR CRITICAL CARE NURSING EDUCATION

No studies were found that addressed the prioritizing of identified learning needs or that described expected outcomes of the educational process.

IMPLEMENTATION OF THE EDUCATIONAL PROCESS

In a 1979 national survey conducted by AACN to describe current practice in critical care areas in United States hospitals, data about staff orientation and in-service education were collected and reported by Sullivan and Breu (1982). In most hospitals with intensive care units (ICUs) orientation was provided for the staff (83%). There was a relationship between hospital size and the provision of orientation for staff, with smaller hospitals less likely than larger hospitals to offer an orientation program specifically for new nurses in critical care units. Regional differences in orientation for ICU nursing staff also were found, with a lower incidence in the West North Central, West Central, and Mountain regions than in other geographic locations.

Most respondents (88%) reported an ongoing in-service educational program for the nursing staff. A correlation was found again between hospital size and the provision of in-service education. Regional differences likewise were noted. Data from a large number of hospitals (78%) indicated that ICU nurses were sent to other institutions for training, though this practice was less likely for hospitals with more than 400 beds. A small number of respondents (23%) reported that they trained nursing staff from other institutions, and those training hospitals tended to be large institutions. Further description of the orientation and in-service education programs was not reported.

Gottschall, Bennetta, Klee, and McFarland (1983) surveyed 28 hospitals in one state to determine what was being offered in educational orientation programs for critical care nurses. Formal programs were offered by 54% of the respondents, whereas 13% offered only on-the-job training. Thirty-three percent reported that both formal and informal programs were offered. A wide range of classroom and clinical hours were reported. Program frequency ranged from 1 to 12 offerings per year, with 54% offering the program 2 to 4 times a year. Number of participants varied, with 50% of the respondents reporting between 11 and 20 participants. Faculty–participant ratio for clinical experience ranged from 1:1 to 1:11. Program planners included ICU head nurses (16%) and clinical specialists (20%), wheres none of the respondents reported that ICU staff nurses participated in program planning. The *Core Curriculum for Critical Care Nursing* (Borg, Nikas, Stark, & Williams, 1981) was used as a blueprint by 54% of the respondents; 29% required specific texts; and 75% provided a bibliography. The "buddy system" was used as a clinical teaching strategy by 88% of the respondents. Participants were regarded as part of the staffing pattern during orientation by only 12% of the respondents. Almost all of the programs (96%) utilized testing as an evaluation strategy, but only 48% used the test grade to determine whether an orientee would be assigned to the ICU on a permanent basis.

Hansell and Foster (1980) investigated an alternative to classroom teaching. Test scores of nonrandomly assigned orientees receiving a structured classroom teaching program were compared to those receiving self-instructional modules. Investigators were not blind to group assignment. Tests were administered before and after a 3-week orientation to 12 nurses in the control group and 12 nurses in the experimental self-instructional group. Although scores on the pretest were similar for both groups, the self-instructional group scored higher on the posttest and had a greater mean change in score; these differences were not statistically significant at the 0.05 level. An additional finding was that head nurse appraisals at 3 months indicated a greater satisfaction with the performance of nurses in the experimental group. Mean completion time and mean scores for each area of the self-instructional modules were examined, and the investigators found that the greatest amount of learning occurred in the area of gastroenterology, whereas the cardiovascular area, particularly electrocardiography, required the most time. Significant reductions in costs were reported with the self-instructional modules as well as greater orientee satisfaction. Hansell and Foster sought to compare strategies for teaching critical care nursing content and skills, but the findings are limited by the nonrepresentative sample, the inability to remain blind to group assignment, and the variation among subjects relative to the study variables.

Fenn and Fassel (1979) investigated the usefulness of videotape presentations as teaching adjuncts in continuing education for critical care nurses. Ten nurses were assigned either to a videotape group ($n = 5$) or a lecture group ($n = 5$), and a control group of 7 non-ICU nurses was matched with the videotape or lecture groups on the basis of the Otis Self-Administering Tests of Mental Ability (Otis, 1956). Clinical pulmonary physiology was selected as the subject matter. Construct validity and test–retest reliability were examined for the 54-item test prior to administration to the three groups. The test was administered immediately following the learning experience and again 10 days later. No significant difference was found between videotape and lecture group scores at posttest and follow-up.

Teaching nurses to set priorities for patients with pain resulting from acute myocardial infarction was the focus of a study reported by Riegel and Dracup (1986). They hypothesized that educating critical care nurses in stress theory would raise the priority the nurses gave to pain intervention for patients with acute myocardial infarction. Nurses were assigned randomly to the experimental ($n = 43$) or the control ($n = 59$) group. The experimental group intervention consisted of a 2-hour scripted class; the control group received no intervention. An instrument was developed to measure the priority given to various nursing interventions, including pain relief in response to a series of 12 simulated clinical case studies. Content validity was determined by a panel of experts. The priority for pain relief scores of the experimental group on the first posttest and on the final posttest was significantly higher than similar scores for the control group. Although the authors acknowledged that the findings did not mean that changes in actual practice occurred, they suggested that such an outcome might be possible.

Only 3 experimental studies were found in which investigators addressed the implementation of instructional strategies. Small sample sizes and inability to control intervening variables set limits on the generalizability of the findings.

EVALUATION OF THE EDUCATIONAL PROCESS

Houser (1977) reported an evaluative study designed to identify predictors of performance levels in special care units. Fifty subjects were studied at three different time intervals following employment to determine if successful job performance could be predicted on the basis of postorientation test scores, type of basic nursing education program, prior clinical experience, or time for adaptation to employment in the special care unit. The author concluded that test scores must be considered as only one factor in predicting a successful performance. High or very low scores tended to be more predictive of performance than scores in the middle range. Basic educational program was a predictor for only the associate degree graduate, with

100% of the associate degree graduates exhibiting low performance levels. Prior clinical experience, either in a special care unit or elsewhere, was a predictor of successful job performance. Although performance scores at the 3-month interval were low for subjects regardless of test scores and prior clinical experience, adaptation to the role of critical care nurse was apparent at the 6-month interval for the majority of subjects. The findings are limited by the small, nonrepresentative sample and by the absence of validity and reliability data for the examinations and the performance scales.

Stross and Bellfy (1979) surveyed a group of coronary care nurses attending a continuing education program to determine their perceptions of their initial training and ongoing continuing education in coronary care. Two hundred completed questionnaires were received (94%), the results indicating that 81% (162 of 200) had completed formal training in coronary care nursing. Sixty-five percent of this group reported that their initial training adequately prepared them for their duties. Only 42% were required to complete successfully an examination of competency prior to beginning work. Subjects also were asked to rate their ability to identify heart murmurs on a 5-point scale. When the ratings were compared to actual test results, the investigators concluded that the nurses had accurate perceptions of their abilities. However, insufficient information was provided regarding the test administered to judge the accuracy of the conclusion.

The paucity of studies related to evaluation of the education process in critical care nursing precluded any conclusions about the realization of desired outcomes. Additionally, studies addressing the educational process were based on small, nonrepresentative samples and measured dependent variables with instruments with questionable validity and reliability. Confounding variables seldom were controlled or addressed.

FACTORS INFLUENCING CRITICAL CARE NURSING EDUCATION

No studies were identified that addressed institutional, professional, or individual factors influencing the provision of critical care nursing education.

CONCLUSIONS

The research literature that is focused on critical care nursing education is sparse. Lists of educational needs have been generated, but they remain unsupported by empirical research data. One instrument is available to test basic knowledge in critical care nursing. Learning needs have not been prioritized, and expected outcomes from the educational process have not been described.

The incidence of in-hospital orientation and educational programs has been reported, as well as some descriptive information regarding offerings. A small number of studies addressing teaching strategies have been reported, but limitations preclude generalizability. No conclusions can be reached relative to outcomes of critical care nursing education, nor can factors affecting the educational process be described systematically.

RECOMMENDATIONS FOR FUTURE RESEARCH

The small number of investigators examining critical care nursing education suggests that research related to all aspects of the educational process is warranted. The conceptual model that served as the framework for this review offers some directions for this research.

The base of general education upon which specialty education rests should be examined to determine what knowledge, skills, and attitudes are present upon entry into the specialty. Predictor variables then could be discovered and used to plan educational strategies for nurses differing in assessment parameters. Attention must be directed toward the development of valid and reliable methods of assessing the learning needs of nurses entering the specialty.

The *Education Standards for Critical Care Nursing* (Alspach, Bell, et al., 1986) draw attention to the procedural and structural elements of the educational process and detail the elements of an educational process that require study. Administrative framework and human and nonhuman resources all are believed to be influential in the educational process, but their impact largely is undocumented and warrants investigation. Little is known about the processes of assessment, planning, implementation, and evaluation. A relationship between these processes and the provision of quality patient care is inferred from the model, but documentation is lacking. Finally, demonstration projects are needed to document the contribution of various elements of the educational standards in achieving the desired outcome of quality patient care.

REFERENCES

American Association of Critical Care Nurses. (1984). *Definition of critical care nursing.* Newport Beach, CA: Author.

Alspach, J. G. (1983, November). *Issues in critical care education.* Key address presented at AACN Leadership Institute, Chicago, IL.

Alspach, J. G., Bell, L., Canobbio, M. M., Christoph, S. B., Kahn, R. C., Roberts, W. L., Turzan, L., & Weincek, C. (1986). *Education standards for critical care nursing.* St. Louis, MO: Mosby.

Alspach, J. G., & Williams, S. W. (1985). *Core curriculum for critical care nursing* (3rd ed.). Philadelphia, PA: Saunders.

Bertram, D. (1982). The concept of critical care nursing. *Focus on AACN, 9*(1), 5.

Borg, N., Nikas, D., Stark, J., & Williams, S. (1981). *Core curriculum for critical care nursing* (2nd ed.). Philadelphia, PA: Saunders.

Canfield, A. (1981). Clinical competencies for critical care nurses. *Western Journal of Nursing Research, 3,* 272–279.

Canfield, A. (1982). Controversy over clinical competencies. *Heart & Lung, 11,* 197–199.

Day, H. W. (1963). Preliminary studies of an acute coronary care area. *Lancet, 83,* 53–55.

Disch, J. (1980). Scope of practice defined. *Focus on AACN, 7*(3), 18.

Fenn, J., & Fassel, B. (1979). Research in critical care nursing education: Production of videotapes for in-hospital use. *Heart & Lung, 8,* 313–317.

Gottschall, M. A., Bennetta, P., Klee, S., & McFarland, G. (1983). Critical care orientation programs. *Nursing Management, 14*(10), 32–34.

Hansell, H. N., & Foster, S. B. (1980). Critical care nursing orientation: A comparison of teaching methods. *Heart & Lung, 9,* 1066–1072.

Houser, D. M. (1977). A study of nurses new to special care units. *Supervisor Nurse, 8*(7), 15.

Jackle, M., Ceronsky, C., & Petersen, J. (1977). Nursing students' experience in critical care: Implications for staff development. *Heart & Lung, 6,* 685–690.

Meltzer, L. E. (1965). Coronary units can help decrease deaths. *Modern Hospital, 104*(1), 102–104.

Otis, A. S. (1956). *Otis self-administering tests of mental ability.* New York: Harcourt Brace Jovanovich.

Petersen, J., Jackle, M., & Ceronsky, C. (1977). Nursing students' experience in critical care. *Journal of Nursing Education, 16*(7), 3–9.

Riegel, B. J., & Dracup, K. (1986). Teaching nurses priority setting for patients with pain of acute myocardial infarction. *Western Journal of Nursing Research, 8*, 306–320.

Roberts, W. L., Alspach, J. G., Canobbio, M. M., Christoph, S. B., Kuhn, R. C., Turzan, L., & Weincek, C. (1986). Critical care nursing education: An overview. *Heart & Lung, 15*, 115–126.

Stross, J. K., & Bellfy, L. C. (1979). Continuing education for coronary care nurses. *Heart & Lung, 8*, 318–321.

Sullivan, S., & Breu, C. (1982). Survey of critical care nursing practice. Part IV. Staffing and training of intensive care unit personnel. *Heart & Lung, 11*, 232–247.

Thierer, J., Perhus, S., McCracken, M. L., Reynolds, M. A., Holmes, A. M., Turton, B., Berkowitz, D. S., & Disch, J. M. (Eds.). (1981). *Standards for nursing care of the critically ill.* American Association of Critical Care Nurses. Reston, VA: Reston Publishing.

Torrez, M. R. (1972). Educational needs of the coronary care nurse. *Heart & Lung, 1*, 254–262.

Toth, J. C. (1984). Evaluating the use of the Basic Knowledge Assessment Tool (BKAT) in critical care nursing with baccalaureate nursing students. *Image: The Journal of Nursing Scholarship, 16*, 67–71.

Toth, J. C., & Ritchey, K. A. (1982). News from nursing research: The Basic Knowledge Assessment Tool (BKAT) for critical care nursing. *Heart & Lung, 13*, 272–279.

Chapter 8

Nursing Research Education

JoAnn S. Jamann-Riley
School of Nursing
Columbia University

CONTENTS

Undergraduate and Graduate Content
Teaching Strategies
Curriculum Structure
Doctoral Education
Research Education in Action
    Research Centers
    Postdoctoral Education
Future Directions

In the past three decades nursing leaders have made a concerted effort to establish a foundation of nursing research. Before midcentury the base of nursing practice and understanding was drawn largely from tradition and experience. Nurse leaders began in the 1950s to develop strategies to introduce research content into all levels of nursing education. Most of these historical developments, such as federal funding for graduate education, establishment of research journals, and the formation of research committees and councils, are known. The focus of this chapter is on current practices in research education and identification of trends that can shape educational practices in the 1990s.

A MEDLINE search of the English literature, 1982 through 1987, was done, using the indicators of education–nursing and research. Through the computer search 167 articles in 26 journals were identified. An index search was completed of four journals for the years 1980 through 1987, *Journal of Nursing Education, Nursing Research, Research in Nursing and Health,* and *Western Journal of Nursing Research,* and of the *Journal of Professional Nursing* for 1985 through 1987.

Of the articles reviewed, only 21 were research reports. Most were studies of teaching strategies and generally were weak methodologically. A few studies of the levels of content and curriculum structure were found. However, the bulk of the information shared through publication came from the experience and judgment of nurses whose practice encompassed some degree of research education. In this chapter a synthesis of research findings is reported. The aim is to sharpen the issues and gain an organizing perspective from which substantive studies in research education may be drawn.

UNDERGRADUATE AND GRADUATE CONTENT

Because research has been incorporated at all levels of education, several investigators conducted surveys to determine the patterns and content that were being included. Shelton (1979) gathered data from 216 National League for Nursing (NLN)-accredited baccalaureate programs. Of the programs responding, 31% had a required research methods course in the curriculum, and 65% indicated that research content was integrated into other undergraduate courses. The major outcomes expected from these learning experiences were that students would be able to discover problems, test hypotheses, use the problem-solving method, critique research reports, and apply findings to their practices.

In 1980, two surveys, using essentially the same sampling population as Shelton, were reported in which the rapid inclusion of research as part of undergraduate nursing education was demonstrated. Spruck (1980) surveyed 286 NLN-accredited baccalaureate programs. Of the 263 schools that responded, 64% reported a required course in research, and 1% indicated that an elective research course was available. Furthermore, the respondents indicated that most students had positive attitudes toward research and that exceptional students were encouraged to pursue graduate study. Thomas and Price (1980) reported that 198 of the 205 respondents to their survey of 291 NLN-accredited baccalaureate programs reported courses in research. The findings indicated that the aim of this level of research education was to prepare consumers of research.

Murdaugh, Kramer, and Schmalenberg (1981) queried 70 schools of nursing with both undergraduate and graduate programs. The investigators received responses from 41 schools, 16 of which had doctoral programs in nursing. Of the 41 schools reporting, 75% had courses at the graduate level. Research methods courses were a part of the program of study in all of the masters programs, and all doctoral candidates were required to complete a dissertation.

No other investigations of the inclusion of research content in nursing education were located in the literature. However, several authors expressed their expectations for research education. Fawcett (1985) gave a clear typology for nursing education programs based on the expectations of graduates from the various levels of nursing education. Fontes (1986) indicated that the most important question is what content to include at each level. She affirmed a consensus that the doctoral level is the most appropriate for preparing independent investigators, but much confusion remains for other levels of preparation and practice. Snyder-Halpern (1984) contended that doctoral preparation in nursing should not be limited to nursing science. Recognizing that preparation for clinical nursing research is extremely important, she made a case for retaining support for nurses to study at the doctoral level in other disciplines. Research education attained in other disciplines enriched and cross-fertilized ideas, theories, and approaches of nursing investigations.

Virtually no other studies have been published on research education at the graduate level. Murphy (1984) reviewed the content of the 136 papers presented at the First Annual Scientific Meeting of Research in Nursing Education, held in January 1983, and found that only five papers addressed graduate education.

TEACHING STRATEGIES

In 1984 de Tornyay reviewed the research literature, 1971 to 1982, on the teaching–learning process in nursing education. Her review supported the observation that very little attention was paid to research education at the graduate level. Of the 37 studies de Tornyay selected to review, only 6 had graduate students as subjects. She expressed concern that many of the studies of the teaching–learning process lacked generalizability, had inadequate controls, or had overdrawn conclusions. The same criticisms can be made of the studies reviewed in this report. Regardless, the investigators are to be commended for approaching the critical area of research education and initiating some study of the problems identified therein.

Kramer, Holaday, and Hoeffer (1981) explored the teaching of nursing research at both the undergraduate and graduate levels. The investigators concluded that in comparing teaching strategies small group work was most effective in producing positive attitudes toward nursing research at both levels. Research education at the masters level also was enhanced with student–faculty participation in research activities.

The remainder of the studies on teaching–learning had samples drawn from one institution. Consequently, the findings lacked generalizability. Nonetheless, specific research methods were described, and the results opened avenues for further investigation.

Sakalys (1984) examined the effects of a research methods course on undergraduate students' cognitive development. The sample was comprised of 50 volunteers assigned to two groups, with a research methods course given to one group. Both groups were tested before and after the course. No significant difference in cognitive development was found. Sakalys concluded that an isolated course in research is not likely to develop cognitive processes fundamental to scientific inquiry.

McIntosh and Pettit (1984) offered students an option of two teaching strategies. The students could choose between developing a clinical research proposal or doing a debate. No difference was found in the learning outcomes of participating students. Gohsman (1983), however, found that involving students in faculty research projects generally resulted in favorable student evaluations. Over 2½ years, five groups of students were given the opportunity to participate in 16 hours of research activity during a term. All students who collected data were sent a copy of the faculty member's research report.

Swanson and Kleinbaum (1984) examined students' attitudes toward research before, during, and after the junior and senior years in a baccalaureate nursing program. Although the overall research attitude scores did not change significantly either before or after having a research course, students were more confident in their understanding of research and their belief that research is a responsibility of doctorally prepared nurses. Another interesting finding was that students' interest in graduate study declined from the pretest to the last measure taken in their senior year.

In reviewing the research literature, Overfield and Duffy (1984) found a paucity of research on teaching; nonetheless, a variety of approaches were used to teach research at the baccalaureate level, which they categorized as learning by doing, proposing, or critiquing. All of these approaches still are used, but most of the articles based on experience of teaching nursing research at the baccalaureate level have remained focused on content or attitude change, rather than the learning process. Several articles have been published on experiential methods of learning about research for baccalaureate students, with no formal research reported on these methods. Examples of such articles include Dean (1986), Harris (1986), Johnson (1984), Ludeman (1981, 1982), Muhlenkamp (1981), and Shelley (1983).

Little investigation has been done on the teaching–learning strategies for graduate students in research education. The findings for undergraduate students cannot be extended to graduate students. Graduate students, whose educational and experiential backgrounds, learning goals, and performance expectations differ considerably from those of undergraduates, approach the learning process in research education with diverse attitudes, knowledge, and skills.

Selby and Tuttle (1985) conducted a pilot study with a group of 25 graduate students. Investigator-developed measurement tools for knowledge and attitudes toward research were used before and after a guided design method of instruction. Of the students studied, 71% had a positive change in attitude toward research, 75% had an increased interest in research, and 92% had confidence in their ability to conduct clinical research. This study had a weak design for the investigation of learning strategies appropriate for preparing nurse researchers. However, the authors are to be commended for validating their own practice using the research process and for communicating their findings.

Another study that was addressed to research education at the graduate level was the Conduct and Utilization of Research in Nursing Project. Horsley, Crane, Crabtree, and Wood (1983) had students in group work over 2 semesters. The collegial relationships in the group process of addressing clinical questions facilitated the learning of both seasoned and not-so-seasoned researchers. The positive group work led to fewer false starts and more positive outlooks on conducting and using research. From practical application of these findings, Firlit, Kempt, and Walsh (1986) discussed how to focus the process of conducting research that leads to utilization of research. Building on the work of Horsley et al., they integrated the use of problem solving with the change process by focusing on the student's learning to develop clinical trials.

Several authors reported teaching–learning strategies that had positive outcomes when used with graduate students; these strategies are not supported empirically. For examples, refer to Austin, Opie, and Frazier (1987), Broome and Demi (1987), Perry (1986), Sarkis and Connors (1986), Spratlen (1982), and Warner and Tenney (1985).

CURRICULUM STRUCTURE

A faculty alive with the love and skills of research must have had at least an adequate curriculum, a reasonable environment, and re- sources for research in order to produce a sufficient yield of nurse researchers. In her review of curricular research in nursing, Stember (1984) found that very little research had been done on nursing curricula. She speculated that the lack of socialization of investigators in their training toward publishing accounts in part for the lack of published curricular research. No specific studies of research curricula were found in the present review; however, a few related studies add to knowledge of what has occurred.

Thiele (1984) investigated whether the placement of research in the undergraduate curriculum made a difference. She studied three groups of students in one school over 3 years. A 12-item assessment instrument was administered 2 weeks after the students graduated. One group had a research course in the sophomore year, another in the junior year, and a third in the senior year. Although this study was weak methodologically, the results suggested that early placement was preferable. Those students who had the research course in either the sophomore or junior years scored higher on productivity mea- sures, such as use of refereed journals, positive attitudes toward research, and application to clinical practice.

Graduate nurses have brought to research education a wide variety of knowledge and perceptions about research in the everyday practice of nurses in many settings. Often there have been incongruent expectations between faculty and graduate students. Fugelberry ("On the Scene," 1986) examined nursing research in practice settings and found that most nurses had positive attitudes but did not view research as part of the job. Using a descriptive correlational design, Fugelberry investigated the attitudes of administrators and staff nurses toward nursing research in five community hospitals. She used the Kilian Questionnaire (cited in "On the Scene," 1986) with 118 respondents (45% return) to evaluate attitudes toward, involvement in, and perceived competence for research. Many of the respondents (75%) never had a course in research. This finding alone has implications for continuing research education and collaborative practices in the clinical setting. Careful assessment of graduate curriculum prerequisites also must be considered. Fugelberry found that staff nurses generally were favorable to research but had little involvement. As might be expected, nurses with administrative responsibilities were involved more in research activities than staff nurses. Likewise, the higher the nurse's education the more likely she or he was to be involved in research and to have more positive attitudes.

Attitude formation and socialization into the research component of professional nursing practice received the most emphasis in the literature on research education at the graduate level. Most of the authors based their work on experience and thoughtful analysis. Brogan (1982) studied a group of masters students in one school to determine whether course work in research methods and statistics socialized them into a research role. Two cohorts, 60 in each group, were given self-administered questionnaires during their course of study. Less than 30% expressed interest in doing research in their future practices. Those with the most professional nursing experience expressed the most interest in doing research, both as they entered the courses and when the coursework was completed.

Anderson (1986) investigated the workload of baccalaureate faculty and its impact on research activities. Although her results from three undergraduate faculties cannot be generalized, the results merited consideration in regard to research education. First, the majority of faculty were prepared at the masters level, which did not prepare them to function as independent investigators or as leaders in research development. Second, the academic environment was not conducive to sustained research activity. Anderson found that faculty were dissatisfied and experienced conflict. They expressed desires to have their teaching time reduced and their research time increased. Faculties recognized that research was the most rewarded behavior in the academic setting, but clinical teaching responsibilities inhibited scholarly research.

DOCTORAL EDUCATION

Doctoral-level study is the key to research education to enhance the efforts of practicing nurse researchers and to expand and increase future nursing research productivity. Studies of research productivity of doctorally prepared nurses gave evidence that greater efforts were necessary. In 1983 Brimmer et al. reported a 2-year national study of educational and employment characteristics of doctorally prepared nurses. The data were collected during 1979–80 from 1,964 respondents, 70% of whom had completed doctoral study during the 1970s. Two findings stand out as important indicators for the future. First, over two thirds of the doctorally prepared nurses in the United States were employed by colleges and universities; thus, the expectations of faculty roles and functions need to be examined for research responsibilities and implementation. Second, the typical nurse received a doctoral degree at about age 40, which is much later than in most other disciplines. Consequently, both work and career patterns need to be studied to incorporate realistic expectations to extend the contributions of doctorally prepared nurses.

The research environments of doctoral programs do not account for the low level of research productivity of their graduates. Holzemer and Chambers (1986) reported that most faculty members in doctoral programs perceived the environments and resources as excellent for research production. The most significant standard for assessing quality of doctor programs was the scholarship of the faculty as measured by quantity and quality of research publications, funding secured, faculty ranks attained, and professional leadership positions assumed. Students assessed the academic research experience as most positive with associate professors. However, there was an inverse relationship between quality of the academic environment and alumni productivity. Doctoral programs may have been good models, but positive research environments were not the norm for most colleges. No doubt the employment environment had a very strong impact on research productivity.

RESEARCH EDUCATION IN ACTION

Resolution of controversies, such as qualitative versus quantitative methods, clinical versus basic research, and independent versus collaborative research education, have led nursing leaders to focus their energies and resources on positive research education and practice actions. Concentration of research personnel and resources in both academic and service agencies has led to new environments in which novice and experienced nurse researchers can learn and practice.

Research Centers

Discrepancies between the ideal and the real disappear when cohorts of nurse researchers and practitioners work together to create a climate for serious inquiry into nursing problems. Pranulis and Gortner (1985) identified the elements for a productive research environment as organizational emphasis and support, resources, administrative support, and conducive social climate. These elements have been developed in a variety of agencies.

A few examples of nursing research centers are described in the literature. Gortner (1985) outlined the development of such a center at the University of California at San Francisco. A 5-year plan was executed through faculty development, a peer-review committee, internal funding, and a research emphasis grant for doctoral programs from the federal government. This center nurtured faculty research throughout the calendar year, which has benefitted beginning researchers who either were faculty members or graduate students of nursing. Ozbolt (1986) discussed how nursing research was promoted through the Center for Nursing Research at the University of Michigan. These two case studies gave in-depth comprehensive information that could be used for replication. Many other universities with doctoral programs in nursing have created research centers to facilitate both student and faculty research but have not published reports on the developmental process.

Concurrent with the development of research centers in schools of nursing was the development of clinical nursing research programs in nursing service agencies. Hunt et al. (1983) outlined the managerial strategy used in three teaching hospitals in Boston to develop research within a service setting. The goals were to (a) provide a bond for professional growth; (b) reinforce and refine nursing research knowledge; (c) clarify research standards of practice; (d) share instruments, methods, and strategies; and (e) provide a creative outlet for nurse researchers (p. 27). Another advantage of this research network was that it provided educational offerings, both to learn research and to incorporate research findings into practice. This case study included a description of the process, but detailed analysis was lacking. One example of collaborative research was given.

Not all nursing research centers have been located in large metropolitan areas. Mackay, Grantham, and Ross (1984) discussed their experience in building a hospital nursing research department in Halifax, Nova Scotia. They reviewed the process and cited a few of the problems. The planning, resources, implementation strategy, financing, and maintenance of the research program were reported. However, the depth expected in a case-study analysis was lacking.

A study of clinical nurse researchers reported in 1986 by Hagel, Kirchhoff, Knafl, and Bevis confirmed that organizational considerations such as reporting to the chief nurse executive officer and having a sufficient budget were essential to the success of the research program. After surveying the literature to identify important issues for clinical nurse researchers, Hagel and her colleagues conducted telephone interviews with 34 clinical nurse researchers. Their results compared favorably with those issues described in the literature. For example, doctoral preparation was considered a must. The respondents believed that substantial clinical experience along with a sound research background was necessary. Although two thirds had previous teaching experience, it was not perceived to be essential in fulfilling the responsibilities of clinical nurse researchers, which included research education for practitioners and students of nursing.

Postdoctoral Education

No research on postdoctoral research education was found in the literature review. Only within the past decade have any significant efforts been made to make postdoctoral education a reality within the realm of nursing science. Most established nurse researchers recognized and advocated postdoctoral study for nurse scientists to extend the depth of their knowledge and research skill either in an area of specialization or in a basic science. Other opportunities such as the

Robert Wood Johnson Foundation Clinical Scholars Program have been made available for doctorally prepared nurses to broaden their knowledge and sharpen their skills in clinical nursing research. With more nurses applying for and receiving postdoctoral research fellowships and training awards, postdoctoral study for nurse researchers is becoming an expectation within the profession. The doctoral degree no longer is considered terminal education for nurse researchers.

FUTURE DIRECTIONS

Research is a content area for formal study and an integral force in the development of nursing science and the profession of nursing. Organizing perspectives are required for the systematic investigation of issues and practices in research education. A framework is needed to explore, describe, test, and validate its critical areas. The critical areas gleaned from the literature review include gradual skill development, collaboration, and holistic approaches.

There is a continuum of personal and professional development in research education that is essential for the production of committed and competent nurse researchers. Increasing skill attainment is a sound developmental principle and an essential responsibility to be implemented for developing the science and improving the practice of nursing. This continuum of experience should permit the student of nursing research to go the full extent from neophyte to mentor.

The typology developed by Fawcett (1985) can serve as a common progressional model for content presentation and experiential learning. In her model Fawcett addresses research generation, dissemination, and the use of the research process and findings. Both cross-sectional and longitudinal studies using this model can shed light on the critical process elements and actual outcomes at each level of research education in nursing.

Intersecting the continuum of skill development and role implementation are critical learning elements identified by Kim (1984) as orientation toward research; knowledge of process and methods; skill, attitudes, and established outcomes. The relationships among any or all of these variables are fertile avenues of investigation.

An expanded vision of the context in which nursing research can be pursued opens many possibilities for research education in nursing. Creativity in research designs, better use of resources, and wider generalizations emerge when collaborative research efforts are made. Collaboration facilitates the sharing of knowledge, optimal use of expertise, and maximal use of resources. Whether the collaboration is complementary, supplementary, or mentorship, the potential outcomes are increased productivity and stronger conclusions. Major advantages of collaborative research are reinforced enthusiasm for the investigation, possibly more complex designs, larger data bases, broader generalizations, and better dissemination of the findings. Faculty–student collaboration provides learning opportunities along the continuum of skill development in all of the critical elements. Service–education collaboration opens the door to defining nursing research problems with clinical relevance and increases the potential for implementation of research findings, replication of studies, and ongoing validation of nursing practice.

The concept of holism in nursing embraces not only the holistic practice of nursing (body, mind, and spirit) and the unification of the functions of professional practice (service, education, and research), but also comprehensiveness in these dimensions. There has been an increasing tolerance of viewing nursing from other perspectives or combining nursing with other scientific and practice disciplines. Also, nurses have been encouraged to study in other disciplines to expand the boundaries of nursing practice and to multiply the research orientations and repertoire for nursing science. Inclusion of students in interdisciplinary experiences can broaden their knowledge base, expand their professional relationships, and increase their communication skills. Their intellectual horizons can be heightened and intellectual curiosity peaked.

Triangulation of research methods can increase the depth of understanding complex nursing problems. Consequently, students of nursing research should strive continually to expand their perspectives and skills, whether they are beginning or seasoned nurse researchers. Interdisciplinary education and triangulation are but two of the emerging possibilities for adding comprehensiveness to nursing research education.

Investigations of nursing research education are sparse. The few studies reported are weak methodologically and lack a research framework. In the present review of research, trends that shape research education practices have been identified as well as elements for developing a conceptual framework for investigating nursing research education.

REFERENCES

Anderson, M. A. (1986). BSN faculty workload. Its impact on research. *Nursing Outlook, 34,* 199.

Austin, J. K., Opie, N. D., & Frazier, H. A. (1987). Strategy for teaching evaluation research in psychiatric/mental health nursing. *Journal of Nursing Education, 26,* 108–112.

Brimmer, P. F., Skoner, M. M., Pender, N. J., Williams, C. A., Fleming, J. W., & Werley, H. W. (1983). Nurses with doctoral degrees: Education and employment characteristics. *Research in Nursing and Health, 6,* 157–165.

Brogan, D. R. (1982). Professional socialization to a research role: Interest in research among graduate students in nursing. *Research in Nursing and Health, 5,* 113–122.

Broome, M. E., & Demi, A. S. (1987). Strategies for teaching nursing research: Teaching statistical analysis—a computer application activity. *Western Journal of Nursing Research, 9,* 132–137.

Dean, P. G. (1986). Strategies for teaching nursing research: Participant observation. *Western Journal of Nursing Research, 8,* 378–382.

de Tornyay, R. (1984). Research on the teaching–learning process in nursing education. *Annual Review of Nursing Research, 2,* 193–210.

Fawcett, J. (1985). A typology of nursing research activities according to educational preparation. *Journal of Professional Nursing, 1*(2), 75–78.

Firlit, S. L., Kemp, M. G., & Walsh, M. (1986). Strategies for teaching nursing research: Preparing master's students to develop clinical trials. *Western Journal of Nursing Research, 8,* 106–109.

Fontes, H. (1986). Stratifying research curricula—The logical next step. *Nursing and Health Care, 7,* 258–262.

Gohsman, B. (1983). Strategies for teaching nursing research: Involving students in faculty research. *Western Journal of Nursing Research, 5,* 250–253.

Gortner, S. R. (1985). The University of California at San Francisco research environment. *Western Journal of Nursing Research, 7,* 387–389.

Hagel, M. E., Kirchhoff, K. T., Knafl, K. A., & Bevis, M. E. (1986). The clinical nurse researcher: New perspectives. *Journal of Professional Nursing, 2*(5), 282–286.

Harris, S. L. (1986). Development of computer assisted instruction. Lessons for teaching nursing research. *Computers in Nursing, 4,* 140, 182.

Holzemer, W. L., & Chambers, D. B. (1986). Healthy nursing doctoral programs: Relationship between perceptions of the academic environment and productivity of faculty and alumni. *Research in Nursing and Health, 9,* 299–307.

Horsley, J. A., Crane, J., Grabtree, M., & Wood, D. (1983). *Using research to improve nursing practice: A guide.* New York: Grune & Stratton.

Hunt, V., Stark, J. L., Fisher, F., Hegedus, K., Joy, L., & Woldrum, K. (1983). Networking: A managerial strategy for research development in a service setting. *Journal of Nursing Administration, 13*(7–8), 27–32.

Johnson, J. M. (1984). Strategies for teaching nursing research: Strategies for including statistical concepts in a course in research methodology for baccalaureate nursing students. *Western Journal of Nursing Research*, *6*, 259–264.

Kim, H. S. (1984). Critical contents of research process for an undergraduate nursing curriculum. *Journal of Nursing Education, 23*, 70–72.

Kramer, M., Holaday, R., & Hoeffer, B. (1981). The teaching of nursing research. Part II: A comparison of teaching strategies. *Nurse Educator, 6*(2), 30–37.

Ludeman, R. (1981). Strategies for teaching nursing research: Experiential learning in data collection. *Western Journal of Nursing Research, 3*, 249–251.

Ludeman, R. (1982). Strategies for teaching nursing research: Experiential learning in data analysis. *Western Journal of Nursing Research, 4*, 124–126.

MacKay, R. C., Grantham, M. A., & Ross, S. E. (1984). Building a hospital nursing research department. *Journal of Nursing Administration, 14*(7–8), 23–27.

McIntosh, D., & Pettit, L. S. (1984). Research proposals and debates: A teaching strategy. *Nursing and Health Care, 5*, 327–329.

Muhlenkamp, A. F. (1981). Strategies for teaching nursing research: Desensitization of the research phobia: Instructor as therapist. *Western Journal of Nursing Research, 3*, 305–309.

Murdaugh, C., Kramer, M., & Schmalenberg, C. E. (1981). The teaching of nursing research: A survey report. *Nurse Educator, 6*(1), 28–35.

Murphy, S. A. (1984). Editorial: Approaches to research in graduate education. *Journal of Nursing Education, 23*, 97.

On the scene: Research as component of graduate study in nursing administration at the University of Washington School of Nursing. (1986). *Administration Quarterly, 11*(1), 27–71.

Overfield, T., & Duffy, M. E. (1984). Research on teaching research in the baccalaureate nursing curriculum. *Journal of Advanced Nursing, 2*(2), 189–196.

Ozbolt, J. G. (1986). Promoting nursing research: The Center for Nursing Research at the University of Michigan. *Western Journal of Nursing Research, 8*, 124–127.

Perry, P. A. (1986). Strategies for teaching nursing research: Integration of research in graduate clinical course. *Western Journal of Nursing Research, 5*, 469–472.

Pranulis, M. F., & Gortner, S. R. (1985). Characteristics of productive research environments in nursing. *Western Journal of Nursing Research, 7*, 128–131.

Sakalys, J. A. (1984). Effects of an undergraduate research course on cognitive development. *Nursing Research, 33*, 290–295.

Sarkis, J. M., & Connors, V. L. (1986). Nursing research: Historical background and teaching information strategies. *Bulletin of the Medical Library Association, 74*, 121–125.

Selby, M. L., & Tuttle, D. M. (1985). Teaching nursing research by guided design: A pilot study. *Journal of Nursing Education, 24*, 250–252.

Shelley, S. I. (1983). The IDIR model for faculty research with students. *Western Journal of Nursing Research, 5*, 301–312.

Shelton, B. (1979). Research components in baccalaureate programs of nursing. *Journal of Nursing Education, 18*(5), 22–23.

Snyder-Halpern, R. (1984). Doctoral preparation: Is nursing guilty of ethnocentric thinking? *Journal of Nursing Education, 23,* 316–317.

Spratlen, L. P. (1982). Strategies for teaching nursing research: Using secondary data in needs assessment approach to nursing assessment. *Western Journal of Nursing Research, 4,* 324–328.

Spruck, M. (1980). Teaching research at the undergraduate level. *Nursing Research, 29,* 251–259.

Stember, M. L. (1984). Curricular research in nursing. *Annual Review of Nursing Research, 2,* 239–262.

Swanson, I., & Kleinbaum, A. (1984). Attitudes toward research among undergraduate nursing students. *Journal of Nursing Education, 23,* 380–386.

Thiele, J. (1984). Strategies for teaching nursing research: Placement of research: Does it make a difference? *Western Journal of Nursing Research, 6,* 356–358.

Thomas, B., & Price, M. (1980). Research preparation in baccalaureate nursing education. *Nursing Research, 29,* 259–261.

Warner, S., & Tenney, J. W. (1985). Strategies for teaching nursing research: A test of computer-assisted instruction in teaching nursing research. *Western Journal of Nursing Research, 7,* 132–134.

PART IV

Research on the Profession of Nursing

Chapter 9

Acquired Immunodeficiency Syndrome

JOAN G. TURNER

SCHOOL OF NURSING
UNIVERSITY OF ALABAMA AT BIRMINGHAM

CONTENTS

Recently, Larson (1988) conducted a systematic review of the previous 52 months of nursing literature in 46 different English-language journals and found 169 articles in which some aspect of acquired immunodeficiency syndrome (AIDS) was discussed. In analysis of these articles, Larson found that 24% were related to some aspect of nursing care and 22% were related to public policy issues; none contained reports of nursing research.

In contrast, 46% of the 481 articles retrieved from the medical literature for a 6-month period in 1986 were reports of related research. Physicians focused primarily on issues related to descriptive

The author gratefully acknowledges the contributions of Patricia A. O'Leary, M.S.N., R.N., doctoral fellow at the School of Nursing, University of Alabama at Birmingham, in the shaping of this review.

epidemiology, pathology, and complications associated with AIDS-related illnesses in their research reports.

The point Larson (1988) made so eloquently is that nursing research necessarily differs from research conducted by other health care professionals such as physicians. Because nursing is unique among the health care disciplines, reports of AIDS-related nursing research are needed to provide an empirical basis for the multiplicity of nursing interventions that are directed at prevention, control, and management of human immunodeficiency virus (HIV) infections in the individual.

The purpose of this review is to present the findings of a concerted attempt to analyze the quantity and quality of nursing research focused on some aspect of HIV infection or AIDS-related diseases. Because Larson's literature search extended through March 1987, particular emphasis was placed on the time period of March 1987 through November 1988.

METHODS OF REVIEW

An initial computer search (MEDLINE) was conducted using the headings *acquired immunodeficiency syndrome*, *AIDS-related disorders or conditions*, and *human immunodeficiency virus infections*. The results were disappointing, as only two citations were found, so a manual search was initiated using the *Index Medicus* and the *Cumulative Index of Nursing and Allied Health Literature* from 1985 to November 1988. An additional manual search was conducted of each issue of *Advances in Nursing Science*, *Nursing Research*, and *Western Journal of Nursing Research* for the same time periods.

When appropriate titles were located, the article was retrieved and examined to determine whether it met the selection criteria for this review. First, only studies where a nurse assumed a major role as investigator were included, even though the content of research in other fields might have been related closely to nursing research. This limitation reflected an attempt to examine a body of congruent research with direct implication for the discipline of nursing. Second, to be included the article had to qualify as a research report.

Determining whether certain authors were nurses was problematic because the credential registered nurse (R.N.) was not always cited along with higher degrees. Thus it became necessary in several instances to make telephone contact with authors or institutions to verify the authors' credentials. To qualify as a research report, the manuscript had to reflect the five major research elements recommended by Cooper (1982), which were evidence of problem formation, data collection, evaluation, analysis, and interpretation. The scientific merit of each study was reviewed according to criteria elaborated by Duffy (1985).

Sixteen usable manuscripts that met selection criteria were located in 12 different English-language journals. Almost all were published in either 1987 ($n = 5$) or 1988 ($n = 10$). One research report appeared in a 1985 issue of *Hospital and Community Psychiatry*. All but two studies were performed using a descriptive design, and a professional nurse was cited as first author in 12 out of 16 manuscripts.

Ten manuscripts were found in which the researchers focused on the characteristics of care providers, specifically attitudes toward persons with AIDS or HIV infection and knowledge of AIDS-related information. Although each research report reviewed had some discernable design or written format weakness, almost all researchers contributed new information or confirmed existing knowledge relative to nursing management (including prevention and control) of HIV-infected individuals. For example, several researchers conducted studies that revolved around AIDS-related knowledge or attitudes among health care professionals, students, and people who were known to be HIV-infected. Other researchers addressed public policy issues, perceptions, and characteristics of HIV-infected individuals.

MAJOR AIDS-RELATED SUBJECT AREAS

AIDS-Related Knowledge and Attitudes

Nine research reports were located that were focused primarily on AIDS-related attitudes, behavioral intentions, and knowledge levels. The purpose of virtually all these studies was to determine levels of knowledge so that appropriate educational interventions could be designed.

Helgerson, Peterson, and the AIDS Education Study Group (1988) conducted a mail survey of public school students and reported that most respondents were misinformed about the methods of HIV transmission and methods that could be effective in avoiding infection. However, those data were collected in 1986, and it was impossible to ascertain whether the survey findings would be applicable today. Replication of the study would be hindered by the lack of a conceptual framework and operational definitions and the fact that the authors did not report estimates of reliability or validity of the data.

Another group of researchers examined worker knowledge and behavioral intentions toward potentially HIV-infected coworkers (Hansen, Booth, Fawal, & Langner, 1988). Through administration of an investigator-designed instrument to nonrandomized comparison groups, the investigators found that health care workers exhibited more positive behavioral intentions toward HIV-infected coworkers than did either blue- or white-collar non-health care workers. The researchers also found that all workers showed a lack of knowledge relative to modes of transmission of HIV and a distrust for official sources of information like the Centers for Disease Control. For example, one subject wrote, "I know the experts say just blood and semen, but I don't trust that" (p. 282).

A study done by van Servellen, Lewis, and Leake (1988) was essentially a needs assessment for continuing education and was conducted among 3,000 randomly selected California R.N.s. Questionnaires ($n = 1,019$) from R.N.s who currently were practicing clinical nursing were used for analysis. The stated purpose was to ascertain nurses' attitudes, fears, and knowledge related to AIDS so that appropriate continuing education could be designed. The researchers reported that only 11% of the respondents ($n = 122$) were able to distinguish between AIDS-related and unrelated symptoms. No date for data collection was given, and no estimates of validity and reliability were provided. Therefore, it was impossible to know whether the test was too difficult or was administered so early in the course of the epidemic that nurses in general practice were not knowledgeable yet about AIDS-related signs and symptoms.

The research reported by Wilson-Young (1988) was the result of a specially designed attitudinal workshop intended to determine whether participation in such a workshop would be effective in changing negative attitudes toward homosexuality in a group of 22 R.N.s. Using a pretest, intervention, posttest design, Wilson-Young concluded that more than half the sample expressed more positive attitudes toward homosexuality after participating in the workshop. Some who reported no change in attitude expressed a desire to develop more positive attitudes over time. Such conclusions must be interpreted with caution because no control group was utilized and no longitudinal testing was done.

Another group of nurses, Turner, Gauthier, Ellison, and Greiner (1988), concluded their research by questioning whether testing of behavioral intentions might be more meaningful than testing attitudes in conjunction with educational interventions. Subjects in both the control and experimental groups of this quasi-experimental study showed significant increases in general AIDS knowledge and more positive attitudes from pretest to 30-day posttest. Although the experimental group showed a significantly greater shift in positive attitudes than did the control group, the researchers were unable to conclude that the reported change in attitude necessarily would result in a change in behavior or behavioral intention. The main recommendation from the study was to measure knowledge and behavioral intentions in conjunction with educational interventions, rather than studying more general attitudes.

Barrick (1988) conducted a descriptive study to measure the relationship between various caregivers' attitudes toward homosexuality and their willingness to care for persons with AIDS. By using self-administered questionnaires completed by R.N.s, licensed practical nurses (L.P.N.s), licensed psychiatric technicians, and hospital orderlies, the researchers concluded that health care workers with more negative attitudes toward gay men and lesbians were less willing to care for persons with AIDS than those with more positive attitudes. Both instruments were reported to have adequate reliability and validity, but no attempt was made to obtain a representative sample of health care workers. No significant differences in attitudes were found between L.P.N.s and R.N.s.

In the fall of 1986, Lester and Beard (1988) invited 177 baccalaureate nursing students to participate in a survey to explore the students' knowledge, fears, beliefs, and other attitudes regarding AIDS. Students who scored higher on fear also had higher knowledge scores, were more homophobic, and were less willing to care for HIV-infected persons. Further, the overwhelming majority of subjects thought that AIDS patients were entitled to the same care as any other patient, but 49% preferred not to care for persons with AIDS themselves.

Douglas, Kalman, and Kalman (1985) published the earliest research that met study criteria. Their instruments consisted of a three-part self-administered tool that included a scale designed to measure homophobia, a demographic information section, and a series of eight questions pertaining to the subject's previous contact with homosexuals. Although multiple design weaknesses were noted, they reported some interesting findings. For example, overall, physicians and nurses scored in the low homophobic range, but males (who were more apt to be physicians) were significantly less homophobic than females (who tended to be R.N.s). Douglas et al. noted that such a finding was in conflict with findings of other researchers, who generally have reported male subjects to be more homophobic than their female counterparts. Additional findings included: (a) Nurses or physicians who had gay or homosexual friends or family members were less homophobic than those without such affiliations, and (b) 31% of subjects reported that they felt more negative about homosexuality since the emergence of AIDS.

Flaskerud (1987) attempted to determine R.N.s' needs for AIDS-related information on a national level for the purpose of developing resources to meet identified needs. She randomly selected 832 nurses from the various council memberships of the American Nurses' Association. The return rate was 62%, and findings were generalized to nurses in the nation at large. One major finding was that a subject's perceived need for AIDS-related information was significantly related to the likelihood of the subject encountering a person with AIDS in the practice setting.

Public Policy Issues

Two studies were located that addressed public policy issues related to AIDS. Mottice, Matsumiya, and Reimer (1987) conducted a survey to determine HIV test criteria and reporting methods for employees and patients in the Veterans' Administration (VA) Medical Center system. Their findings included the following: (a) a trend toward increased patient screening for the HIV antibody in hospitals with higher numbers of cases of AIDS; (b) no specific informed consent policy for HIV testing in the majority of VA medical centers; (c) no counseling prior to testing in 43 of 67 respondent institutions; and (d) HIV testing performed on patients in all reporting facilities, but performed on employees in only 60%.

The second study that was addressed to public policy issues was a mail survey of baccalaureate nursing schools' guidelines and policies regarding AIDS. Bowles and Carwein (1988) received 242 responses

(48% return) from 458 National League for Nursing-accredited bacca-laureate nursing programs and reported that very few schools of nursing had existing guidelines in 1986–1987. Almost half the respondents (49%) said they had no plans to develop a policy to deal with HIV-infected students. Eleven respondents (5%) said they would not let a person with AIDS attend theory classes; 88 (35%) said they would not allow a person with AIDS to attend clinical practicum, and 59 (24%) were undecided.

Perceptions and Characteristics of HIV-Infected Individuals

Three study reports were found that focused on perceptions and characteristics of HIV-infected individuals. Collier et al. (1987) conducted a descriptive study of a convenience sample of 180 homosexual and 26 heterosexual men who were seropositive for the HIV antibody. Their purpose was to determine any relationships between presence of the antibody and cytomegalovirus (CMV), homosexual lifestyle, and T-lymphocyte subset abnormalities among homosexual men. Collier and associates noted that a past history of sexually transmitted diseases was far more common in homosexual men than heterosexual men (86% as compared to 46%), and that the CMV antibody was detected in 96% of homosexual and 50% of heterosexual HIV-infected subjects. Further, there was a statistically significant relationship between CMV seropositivity and T-lymphocyte subset abnormalities among homosexual men, independent of the presence or absence of antibody to HIV. About three quarters of CMV-seropositive homosexual men shed the virus intermittently or continually in semen or urine.

In another descriptive study Rosevelt (1987) examined perceptions of persons with AIDS using a convenience sample of 40 subjects, 20 with AIDS and 20 with AIDS-related complex. The purpose was to describe social support and perceptions of discrimination in the workplace. Subjects were surveyed using two instruments: a standard social support scale and an investigator-designed questionnaire to determine the extent to which discriminatory practices were perceived in the workplace. Reports on measurements of the two main variables were interesting even though the rationale for examining social support in relation to perceived job discrimination was not made explicit. For example, subjects who were employed had significantly lower functional support scores, and the majority of subjects perceived or expressed fear of discriminatory practices in the workplace. However, there were no differences in mean functional support scores for those who did versus those who did not perceive discrimination in the workplace. Finally, gay males scored 25% lower on the social support scale than samples of American men studied previously with the instrument, and friends were perceived as more important sources of support to gay men than were family members.

The third research report that was addressed to characteristics of persons with AIDS was an interdisciplinary study in which a professional nurse was credited as fifth author. Writing with great clarity and detail, Cleary et al. (1988) reported research directed at describing the sociodemographic and behavioral characteristics of persons who were detected as HIV positive when donating blood, had not yet developed AIDS, and were not aware of their infection. For this purpose, 173 subjects whose volunteer blood donations in 1983–1986 routinely were tested for HIV antibody and found positive were obtained over a 10-month period in the New York City area. The researchers described the project as an exploratory study in which information could be obtained that would be useful in developing a randomized, controlled clinical trial of two different programs for providing information, health education, or psychological support to HIV-positive blood donors.

The following findings were reported by Cleary et al. (1988). First, risk factors for HIV infection in this study (and validated by other studies) were one of the following: (a) a sexually active homosexual, (b) a user of illicit intravenous (IV) drugs, or (c) a person with hemophilia. The proportion of women in this study was higher than in similar studies, women accounting for 22% of the total sample of HIV-positive persons compared to roughly 8% in other studies. Another interesting finding that tends to lend credence to bisexuality as a means of HIV spread was that more than half of the homosexual subjects reported heterosexual contacts. In fact, among 104 seropositive men in the sample who reported at least one sexual contact with another man, 62 reported having sexual relations with a woman since 1977 (Cleary et al., 1988).

Most subjects in the Cleary et al. study (1988) were unaware that their blood would be tested for evidence of HIV infection, and written and verbal instructions relative to self-exclusion from blood donation largely went unheeded. The researchers concluded that social pressure to donate, especially in the work setting, was a factor that might encourage high-risk individuals to donate. They recommended that other options should be incorporated into the environment, such as allowing the donor to inform the blood donation facility in confidence either to discard the blood or use it for study purposes only.

Clinical Management of HIV-Infected Individuals

Only two studies were located that related to clinical management of those already HIV-infected. In this case, clinical management might have been directed at preventing further transmission of the virus or at preventing complications by pharmaceutical or other treatment intervention strategies. One such descriptive study was designed using a convenience sample of volunteers in a drug treatment program; 44 of those were seropositive and 137 were seronegative for the HIV antibody. Williams, D'Aquila, and Williams (1987) studied these subjects to determine specific risk behaviors related to seropositivity that might be amenable to educational interventions.

Among the 181 subjects, 24% ($n = 44$) were seropositive at the time of admission into the drug treatment program. There was no significant relationship between sex and seropositivity. Race was the most powerful predictor in that significantly more blacks and Hispanics were seropositive. Subjects reported that they knew about the risk of HIV infection from needles but continued to share them, with many subjects (47%) reporting that they cleaned their "works" with tap water between uses. At the time of data collection in 1986, most subjects did not know about using chlorine solution or alcohol to clean needles and syringes. The mean number of times each subject used a needle for drug injection in a year was 681 times. Overall, IV drug users were conservative sexually in that 22% reported sexual monogamy for the preceding 5-year period; however, the number of sexual partners in the total sample ranged from 1 to 60. In general, subjects showed much less concern about HIV transmission via sexual contact than through the use of contaminated needles (Williams et al., 1987).

The final article reviewed (Jackson et al., 1988) was another interdisciplinary effort in which an experimental design in a longitudinal time frame was used to assess the effect of antiviral therapy on antigenemia, symptoms of HIV-related diseases, various blood cell counts, and prognosis in 16 subjects who were diagnosed with AIDS. Antigenemia, or the level of detectable HIV-antigen in the blood, was used as a dependent variable because it was believed to be a better indicator of viral replication than were other techniques such as viral culturing. The researchers concluded that a dose of zivudine (AZT) at 200 to 250 mg every four hours reduced antigenemia in subjects by 90%. Further, occurrence of zivudine-associated toxicity symptoms requiring a lower dose per 24-hour period was accompanied by increased antigenemia, recurrent symptoms, and decreased immune functioning. Thus, subjects who were unable to tolerate AZT had poorer prognoses than those who could take the drug.

CONCLUSIONS AND RECOMMENDATIONS

The 16 reports reviewed for this chapter represent some progress in nursing's contribution to a research-based body of knowledge relative to AIDS after Larson (1988) was unable to locate a single article some 18 months earlier. However, it must be noted that the comparison is somewhat uneven because the selection criteria were liberalized for this review. For example, to qualify for selection in Larson's study, the first author must have been a professional nurse.

It was not possible to determine how representative these 16 research reports were of nurses' contribution to AIDS-related research. First of all, there is not a standard way to access research reports apart from other published articles, and reports of research are published in some form in most professional nursing and allied health journals. One of the most methodologically tedious steps in this review was systematic scanning of all published works for the time period under consideration and the direct examination of articles whose titles or other publication information suggested that they might be research reports. Factors such as accessibility to any given library's holdings may act to bias retrievability and thereby affect representativeness of the sample.

Another difficulty lay in the attempt to analyze critically the research report form and format. In some journals, such as *Nursing Research* and the *American Journal of Public Health* (*AJPH*), editors have different ways of organizing reports, ostensibly to enhance readability. For example, some publishers have not called for and subsequently published research abstracts, and others do not specify the necessity for a conceptual framework in instructions for manuscript preparation. For example, even though the *AJPH* uses a recognizable research format, instructions for contributors do not mention including a conceptual approach for the study. *Nursing and Health Care* does not publish abstracts with each article. Thus it was often difficult to ascertain whether certain research requisites like operational definitions, abstracts, and conceptual frameworks were part of the original research report.

The great majority of studies were done using a descriptive design (87.5%, $n = 14$). Moreover, the same number were cross-sectional. The researchers focused on AIDS-related knowledge and attitudes, and these studies could be extended using a longitudinal time frame and random samples so that inferences could be drawn about changes that take place over time or in response to educational or personal experiences.

Thus it would appear that nurse researchers need renewed emphasis on both quality and quantity in generating and disseminating AIDS-related research. Serious consideration should be given to the organization of research manuscripts (i.e., questions, conceptual framework, operational definitions, methodology/instrumentation, findings, conclusions, and recommendations). Specific research questions should be posed clearly, and the conceptual framework should be explicit in the design as well as in the analysis and conclusions: Operational definitions should be given for all key variables, and there should be a *critical* review of related literature. In the research reports reviewed for this manuscript, the aforementioned items often were cited as weaknesses, as was the failure of the majority of researchers to report the reliability and validity of instruments used to collect data.

Nurse researchers are urged to examine closely the National Center for Nursing Research priorities listed in Table 9-1 to help them identify the areas in which nursing must establish an empirical knowledge base in order to make substantial contributions to the prevention and management of HIV-related diseases. Taking the 16 research reports reviewed here as an indication of the nursing profession's status on providing that empirical foundation, nurse researchers have begun to prepare for the task. The reality is that the epidemic is growing exponentially both quantitatively and qualitatively in its impact on human potential for health in most parts of the world. AIDS is a human phenomenon, and those affected look to nursing for meaningful intervention strategies; but these strategies would be obscure without the necessary research informational base.

Table 9.1 Topics for Nursing Center Research Within the Priorities Identified by the National Center for Nursing Research

NCNR Priority	Selected Topics
Etiology of AIDS, including identification of predictive factors.	Probability of fetal transmission of HIV from (a) mothers who are HIV positive but asymptomatic and (b) mothers who are HIV positive and have one of the several clinical syndromes associated.
	Incidence of transmission of HIV from transfusion-related cases such as hemophiliacs, particularly among sexual partners.
	Identification of co-factors among high-risk groups that are correlated with increased risk of (a) becoming infected with the HIV virus and (b) developing AIDS.
	Identification of reasons for higher prevalence of AIDS among black and Hispanic populations.
	Correlations of mental, psychological, and behavioral changes with anatomic changes in the brain at autopsy.
Nursing care of AIDS patients at various stages of the disease.	Development of classification system (or testing current systems) for AIDS patients.
	Identification of needs for nursing care based on classification systems.
	Skin care regimens to reduce skin breakdown.
	Nutritional regimens to reduce nausea, vomiting, loss of appetite, diarrhea.
	Trials of various environmental and behavioral manipulations to manage dementias and depression associated with AIDS in various health care settings.
	Differentiation of psychologic, neurologic, and behavioral changes among AIDS patients associated with organic brain changes or with the effects of being chronically ill.
	Assessment of knowledge and attitudes of nurses about AIDS.

Table 9.1   (*continued*)

NCNR Priority	Selected Topics
	Development, implementation, and evaluation of courses to educate nurses and other health care professionals in the care of the AIDS patient.
	Incidence of cross-infection and nosocomial infections among AIDS patients.
	Survey of infection control precautions currently used with AIDS patients.
	Emotional effects on nursing staff of caring for adults/children with AIDS.
Comparative therapeutic and cost effectiveness of nursing interventions in the home, nursing home, and institutional setting.	Survey of patient preferences with regard to delivery of care options during various stages of illness.
	Costs of hospital care for AIDS patients in communities with and without community support groups.
	Identification of support systems and resources in the community necessary to minimize hospital length of stay.
	Effect of availability of third-party reimbursement for home care of AIDS patients.
	Relative costs of nursing care for AIDS patients at all stages of disease in acute care institutions, community-based settings, extended care facilities and/or the home.
	Costs of providing acute care on a unit specified for AIDS patients as compared to caring for patients on general wards.
	Comparison of patient responses and outcomes on these same units.
Knowledge, attitudes, and practices of AIDS patients and effect of AIDS on family functioning.	Effect of HIV infection among asymptomatic individuals on sexual behavior with homosexual partners, with heterosexual partners, with married couples.
	Influence of educational programs on AIDS patients and their family knowledge, attitudes, and adjustment style.

Table 9.1 (*continued*)

NCNR Priority	Selected Topics
	Effect of support groups for significant others on their ability to cope with the needs of the AIDS patient.
	Effect of AIDS on self-concept among children.
	Concerns of parents and siblings of children with AIDS.
	Evaluation of patient wishes regarding life support.
Ethical issues related to diagnosis and treatment strategies.	Impact of HIV antibody status on employment status, particularly in health care settings, the military, and other government or public service jobs.
	Psychological and social impact of HIV-positive status on healthy individuals.
	Changes in the rate of condom use associated with mass media.
Public policy issues, such as methods of early screening and diagnosis and control of spread of the disease.	Effect of education programs (e.g., "safe sex") or other interventions on reproductive and sexual practices of high risk groups.
	The extent of compliance among health care agencies with recommendations published by the Public Health Service and Centers for Disease Control.
	Identification of viable payment alternatives for care of AIDS patients.
	Identification of factors that influence the public to modify high-risk behaviors.
	Assessment of knowledge of preventive strategies for AIDS among high-risk groups, among the general population, among adolescents.
	Evaluation of effectiveness of various methods to provide public education.
	Influence of state or local case finding on the spread of AIDS.

Table 9.1   *(continued)*

NCNR Priority	Selected Topics
	Identification and evaluation of alternative educational and preventive strategies for high-risk groups not reached in the traditional health care system.
Integration of patients, including infants and children in community setting.	School experiences of children with AIDS.
	Effect of educational programs in public schools on children's attitudes and knowledge about AIDS.
	Survey of criteria being used by schools in decisions regarding attendance by children with AIDS.
	Role of the school nurse in educating schoolchildren about AIDS.

REFERENCES

Barrick, B. (1988). The willingness of nursing personnel to care for patients with acquired immune deficiency syndrome: A survey study and recommendations. *Journal of Professional Nursing, 4,* 366–372.

Bowles, C. L., & Carwein, V. C. (1988). Survey of baccalaureate nursing schools' guidelines/policies on AIDS. *Journal of Nursing Education, 27,* 349–353.

Cleary, P. D., Singer, E., Rogers, T. F., Avorn, J., Van Devanter, N., Soumerai, S., Perry, B., & Pindyck, J. (1988). Sociodemographic and behavioral characteristics of HIV antibody-positive blood donors. *American Journal of Public Health, 78,* 953–957.

Collier, A. C., Meyers, J. D., Corey, L., Murphy, V. L., Roberts, P. L., & Handsfield, H. H. (1987). Cytomegalovirus infection in homosexual men. *The American Journal of Medicine, 82,* 593–600.

Cooper, H. M. (1982). Scientific guidelines for conducting integrative research reviews. *Review of Educational Research, 52,* 291–302.

Douglas, C. J., Kalman, C. M., & Kalman, T. P. (1985). Homophobia among physicians and nurses: An empirical study. *Hospital and Community Psychiatry, 36,* 1309–1311.

Duffy, M. E. (1985). A research appraisal checklist for evaluating nursing research reports. *Nursing and Health Care, 6,* 539–547.

Flaskerud, J. H. (1987). Nurses call out for AIDS information. *Nursing and Health Care, 8,* 557–562.

Hansen, B., Booth, W., Fawal, H. J., & Langner, R. W. (1988). Workers with AIDS: Attitudes of fellow employers. *Journal of the American Association of Occupational Health Nurses, 36,* 279–283.

Helgerson, S. D., Peterson, L. R., & the AIDS Education Study Group. (1988). Acquired Immunodeficiency Syndrome and secondary school students: Their knowledge is limited and they want to learn more. *Pediatrics, 81,* 350–355.

Jackson, G. G., Paul, D. A., Falk, L. A., Rubenis, M., Despotes, J. C., Mack, D., Knigge, M., & Emeson, E. E. (1988). Human Immunodeficiency Virus (HIV) antigenemia in the Acquired Immunodeficiency Syndrome (AIDS) and the effect of treatment with zidovudine (AZT). *Annals of Internal Medicine, 108,* 175–180.

Larson, E. (1988). Nursing research and AIDS. *Nursing Research, 37,* 60–62.

Lester, L. B., & Beard, B. J. (1988). Nursing students' attitudes toward AIDS. *Journal of Nursing Education, 27*(9), 399–404.

Mottice, B., Matsumiya, B., & Reimer, L. (1987). Survey on testing criteria and reporting methods for human immunodeficiency virus serologic tests in Veterans Administration Medical Centers. *Infection Control, 8,* 407–411.

Rosevelt, J. (1987). Support for workers with AIDS: Workplace discrimination as perceived by gay men with AIDS or ARC. *Journal of the American Association of Occupational Health Nurses, 35,* 397–402.

Turner, J. G., Gauthier, D. K., Ellison, K. J., & Greiner, D. S. (1988). Nursing and AIDS: Knowledge and attitudes. *Journal of the American Association of Occupational Health Nurses, 36,* 274–278.

van Servellen, G. M., Lewis, C. E., & Leake, B. (1988). Nurses, responses to the AIDS crisis: Implications for continuing education programs. *The Journal of Continuing Education in Nursing, 19,* 4–8.

Williams, A. B., D'Aquila, R. T., & Williams, A. E. (1987). HIV infection in intravenous drug abusers. *Image: Journal of Nursing Scholarship, 19,* 179–183.

Wilson-Young, E. W. (1988). Nurses' attitudes toward homosexuality: Analysis of change in AIDS workshops. *The Journal of Continuing Education in Nursing, 19,* 9–12.

PART V

Other Research

Chapter 10

Interpersonal Communication between Nurses and Patients

BONNIE J. GARVIN
COLLEGE OF NURSING
THE OHIO STATE UNIVERSITY

CAROL W. KENNEDY
COLLEGE OF NURSING
THE OHIO STATE UNIVERSITY

CONTENTS

Many nurse theorists consider the nurse–patient relationship to be a central component in their conceptualizations of nursing. Most theorists and practitioners recognize that the nurse–patient relationship is developed through interaction and is the essence of nursing. Nurse–patient interaction is made possible through communication, a process through which individuals create meaning. Through this communication process the nurse and patient influence one another and the patient's health can be influenced therapeutically and supportively (Kim, 1987).

213

Because communication is an essential part of nursing intervention or serves as the intervention itself, an important part of nursing
research should be focused on understanding the communication
between the nurse and patient and the consequences of this communication for the patient (Diers & Leonard, 1966). Thus the purpose of
this review was to evaluate nursing research related to communication
between nurses and patients. The research was examined as it related
to theory development in the nurse–patient interaction domain of
nursing (Kim, 1987). The current state of development in this domain
reflects activity at the level of concept analysis and some activity at the
level of determining relationships between and among concepts
(Chinn & Jacobs, 1987; Dickoff & James, 1968).

Studies reported in this review were obtained by a MEDLINE
search of nursing journals contained in the *Cumulative Index to
Nursing and Allied Health Literature* and a hand search of the following nursing journals: *Advances in Nursing Science, Journal of International Nursing Studies, Journal of Psychiatric Nursing and Mental
Health Services, Nursing Research, Perspectives in Psychiatric Care,
Research in Nursing & Health*, and *Western Journal of Nursing
Research*. Studies that were conducted in the United States and
reported from 1980 to mid-1989 were included. It is acknowledged
that numerous earlier studies provided the foundation and impetus
for these recent works. Qualifying words used in the search were:
nurse–patient/client, group, and *family*, with the modifiers *interpersonal relationships, communication, therapeutic communication*, and
interaction. Bibliographies were examined for articles missed in the
computer and hand searches. Studies were included that contained
information about the method and results. Theoretical papers and
reviews of the literature were not included.

The focus for the selected studies was nurse–adult patient interpersonal communication. Studies were included if they were focused
on the effect of nurse communication behaviors on the patient or
the effect of patient communication behaviors on the nurse. Studies
also were included if the focus was on nurse or patient communication in actual or potential nurse–patient interactions. Verbal communication behaviors of nurse and patient were included regardless of
whether or not the author made a direct connection to the nurse–
patient relationship.

Studies of personal variables, such as attitudes and personality
traits, were not included unless the investigator examined the relationship of the personal variable to the communication between the

patient and nurse or provided a clear implication for the nurse–patient relationship. Studies of social context, such as organizational climate or cultural beliefs, were not included unless the relationship between the social variables and nurse–patient communication was examined.

In addition, studies were excluded if the focus was on: (a) teaching of interpersonal skills to nurses or students; (b) teaching patients or patient education unless the explicit aim of the study was to examine communication, in which case the communication intervention had to be described; and (c) nonverbal communication, including touch. The last category was excluded because of the recent comprehensive review of this topic in the *Annual Review of Nursing Research* (Weiss, 1988).

Studies of communication in nurse–patient relationships were classified using Kim's (1987) typology of the domains of nursing. The client–nurse domain was one of three domains described. Three components of this domain were client–nurse interaction, client communicative elements, and nurse communicative elements. The terms *client* and *patient* are used throughout this review: the term *client* generally is used to refer to outpatients or healthy subjects, and the term *patient* generally is used when subjects were in hospital settings.

COMMUNICATION IN NURSE–PATIENT RELATIONSHIPS

Although considerable research has been conducted in sociology and psychology on variables that influence interpersonal relationships, little of this work has been transferred to nurse–patient relationships, and even less has been tested empirically. Nursing studies of nurse–patient interaction have covered a wide range of topics. In this section, the organizing topics were empathy, self-disclosure, support, and confirmation.

Empathy

Empathy is recognized as an important concept in the formation of therapeutic relationships and has been studied by many investigators over the past 20 years. Two recent studies are discussed in this section and several more under the section on nurse communicative elements. Studies included here were focused on the effect of nurse empathy on the patient.

Empathy has been defined in a variety of ways by researchers. One way of defining empathy was simply to ascertain that empathy was perceived by the subject. Recent investigators have used Rogers's framework, which holds that the situation not only must be perceived but also must be communicated to the other person (Rogers, 1975). This framework was used by La Monica, Wolf, Madea, and Oberst (1987) to examine the effect of empathy training on outcomes with cancer patients. Using the Empathy Construct Rating Scale (La Monica, 1981), patient-rated nurse empathy and nurse self-report of empathy were high on the pretest. Although the scores did not change significantly after empathy training, patients cared for by nurses in the empathy training group experienced significantly less anxiety and hostility than patients cared for by nurses without empathy training.

In a study also based on Rogers's work that documented perception of clinician empathy in hypertensive and diabetic client groups, Dawson (1985) used the empathy scale of the Barrett-Lennard Relationship Inventory (Gurman, 1977) and found that all 216 subjects perceived low to moderate levels of clinician empathy. Hypertensive subjects perceived less clinician empathy than diabetic and nonchronically ill subjects, and subjects perceived female clinicians to be more empathic than male clinicians. Dawson hypothesized that the failure to perceive clinician empathy might impact on client self-disclosure, but the results did not reveal differences among the groups in self-reported difficulty in disclosing. Dawson suggested that a careful analysis of client–clinician interactions might reveal clinician behaviors that interfere with patient-perceived empathy and self-disclosure.

Self-Disclosure

Self-disclosure is another important concept that has been studied in nurse and patient communication. Based on the writing of Peplau (1975), nurses traditionally have been taught not to disclose personal information. Young (1988) contends that because patient self-disclosure is essential for effective individualized health care, nurses must use communication strategies that facilitate patient self-disclosure. One of these proposed strategies is selective nurse disclosure.

M. N. Johnson (1980) drew on the work of Jourard (1971) and defined self-disclosure as a process of voluntarily revealing information about self to another person (M. N. Johnson, 1980). M. N. Johnson examined self-disclosure between 70 nurses and 68 patients from medical, surgical, psychiatric, and critical care units. A modified version of the Jourard Self-Disclosure Questionnaire (Jourard, 1971) was used for data collection. M. N. Johnson found generally low levels of self-disclosure between nurses and patients across all units. Medical patients had the highest self-disclosure scores, followed by psychiatric patients; surgical and critical care patients had the lowest self-disclosure scores. Surgical nurses had the highest self-disclosure scores, followed by critical care and psychiatric nurses. Medical nurses had the lowest self-disclosure scores. M. N. Johnson offered possible explanations for the low reciprocal disclosure between nurses and patients. These explanations included patient need and nurse role expectations in the particular clinical settings. She suggested that nurses could improve communication with patients by initiating more self-disclosure.

In the study cited earlier on self-disclosure and empathy among hypertensive, diabetic, and nonchronically ill persons, difficulty in disclosing to clinicians was related to the clients' perception of clinician empathy (Dawson, 1985). Clients identified the category of Responses to Health Care as the most important category of self-disclosure, and the Personal Problems and Feelings category was rated as most difficult. Hypertensive clients did not differ from diabetic clients on their reports of difficulty in disclosing; however, hypertensive clients rated the category Responses to Health Care as more important than did the diabetic clients.

In two studies nurses' styles in interactions with clients were described. The investigators concluded that nurses were too structured and task-oriented in their interactions to allow sufficient client self-disclosure. The investigators suggested increased client involvement in nurse–client interactions. In the first study, researchers examined interactions between 35 pediatric nurse practitioners (PNPs) and the mothers of well children (Webster-Stratton, Glascock, & McCarthy, 1986). These investigators did a detailed content analysis of audiotapes of PNPs from 13 states. They used the PNP Interpersonal Behavior Constructs (Webster-Stratton, 1984) in analyzing the tapes and found that the interactions between PNPs and mothers were dominated by PNP questions, commands, and opinions. Rarely was the mother encouraged to ask questions, solve problems, or disclose her knowledge. In addition, the PNPs rarely touched on the emotional aspects of child care. The investigators acknowledged that the PNPs may have been trying to "do their best" for the study, but in the process, they demonstrated social distance and an authoritarian role with their clients.

In the other study, the Bales Interaction Analysis (Bales, 1950) was used to study the interactions of 18 public health nurses and 55 perinatal clients. Morgan and Barden (1985) reported that 54% of the nurses' visits were related to asking for or giving information, while only 8% were described as friendly. Both nurses and clients were uncertain as to whether they had agreed on goals.

In another study, disclosure was defined in reference to revealing information about the client's care. Nurse midwives' disclosure of pain relief practices in nurse–client relationships was examined (Trandel-Korenchuk, 1987). In a model similar to Kim's model (1987), client characteristics, nurse characteristics, and setting characteristics were examined for their impact on the content, method, and timing of nurse disclosures. Questionnaires from 220 nurse midwives, randomly selected from their membership directory, provided the data for the study. The findings gave evidence that the immediate care environment as well as the social environment may have significant effects on the disclosure of information. There was no relationship between client characteristics and the content disclosed by the nurse; however, patient demographic characteristics were related significantly to the method and timing of disclosure by the nurse. The data supported the suggestion that higher education, economic level, and involvement of the patient's spouse/significant other were related to more midwife disclosure.

Whereas nurses obviously must ask clients questions and must give them information, the evidence in the above-described studies suggests a need for more balance between completing what is on the nurse's agenda and allowing an opportunity for clients to share their concerns or questions with the nurse. The above studies show that the concept of self-disclosure is well-defined and that beginning efforts have been made to relate self-disclosure to other concepts.

Support

In another cluster of studies, researchers dealt with supportive behaviors of nurses. Studies were grouped in this category if the primary intent of the investigator was to study some aspect of support. Other studies that included supportive interventions but were focused primarily on another communication concept are discussed elsewhere in this review.

As with many other communication variables, the definition of support in the nursing literature is vague and inconsistent. It is important to distinguish social support from nursing support. Social support includes the idea that a person is part of an ongoing social network involving mutual obligations and material assistance. Nursing support, in contrast, is provided within the nurse–patient relationship. It is limited in time and focused on the patient's concerns. Gardner and Wheeler (1987) designed a study to ascertain patients' perceptions of nursing support and to determine whether patients' perceptions of support differed according to the specialty areas of medicine, surgery, or psychiatry. One hundred and ten patients were interviewed and completed the Supportive Nursing Behavior Checklist, developed by the authors. The 11 categories of nurse support that were identified from the interviews across specialty areas were: being available, promoting comfort, giving information, assisting in expressing feelings, performing specific nursing tasks, helping to solve problems, having a friendly and pleasant attitude, relieving pain, giving reassurance, individualizing care, and touching. The most frequently mentioned item across specialty areas was the nurse being available. The second most frequently assigned category differed among the specialty areas. Patients with medical conditions gave more examples of giving information; those with surgical conditions described behaviors that promoted comfort; and psychiatric subjects more frequently mentioned problem-solving interactions. Interview data correlated favorably with data obtained with the Supportive Nursing Behavior Checklist.

Behaviors that facilitate nurse–patient interactions can be viewed as supportive. In describing nurses' responses that facilitated or inhibited help-seeking behaviors of 40 abused women, Limandri (1987) reported that, among other facilitative behaviors, nurses used active listening and empathizing, suggested tangible resources, avoided telling the woman what to do, and labeled the perpetrator's behavior as abusive. It was important for the nurses to acknowledge the violence and to take an active advocacy role with the woman.

Slavinsky and Krauss (1982) studied outpatient care for the chronically mentally ill. Forty-seven subjects were assigned randomly and treated either through a social approach program run by nurses or a medication clinic supervised by a physician. The nursing treatment was designed to meet needs for both growth and support in regard to dependency and social competence. Patients were encouraged, in group discussions, to seek their own solutions and problems and to explore alternate solutions. After 2 years, contrary to the study hypotheses, the subjects treated only with medication had improved socialization and satisfaction with care ratings and decreased depression and agitation ratings. No differences between groups were reported in hospitalization, days out of the hospital, treatment dropout, symptoms, medication increases, occupation, or satisfaction with their life situation. The investigators suggested several explanations for their findings, including the thoughts that patients may have experienced the supportive treatment as pressure, they may have been encouraged subtly by the nurses to rely too heavily on the mental health system for support, and the nurses may not have expected enough from their patients. The investigators clearly described the difficulties encountered when a researcher implements an interactive treatment, especially over time.

Using nonparticipant observation, two other studies were focused on support and psychiatric patient behavior. In the first study, nursing personnel were found to support deviant behavior and to punish conventional behavior of 44 patients (Simon, Wilson, & Munjas, 1982). Similarly, in the second study they were as likely to reinforce undesirable behavior of 10 patients as to punish it (Niemeier, 1983). Deviant behavior was supported by giving attention to the behavior and illness symptoms. Punishing responses were ignoring the patient and verbalizing disapproval.

Kishi (1983) used content analysis to examine the teaching behaviors of health care providers (four pediatricians and three pediatric nurse practitioners). The investigator found no relationship between the health care providers' affective support and flexibility and client recall of information of 68 mother subjects. Other findings were the lack of a relationship between client recall and (a) the frequency of health care provider questions, (b) the frequency of patient questions, or (c) the amount of client talk. A secondary finding was that white and black mothers enacted different communication patterns; for example, white mothers asked more questions and initiated more talk than black mothers.

Confirmation

Seven studies were categorized under the confirmation concept. The term *confirmation* is a recently developed conceptualization of the qualitative aspects of communication and subsumes other communication variables (Northouse & Northouse, 1985). Confirming communication is reflected when nurses are empathic, disclose their patient-centered thoughts and feelings, and are supportive. The studies in this section essentially portrayed the nurse–patient interaction as one in which the patient is recognized, acknowledged, and endorsed (Laing, 1969). Confirming approaches were contrasted with those that were disconfirming. *Disconfirmation* is communication that fails to recognize the importance of the patient, his or her concerns, or the relationship between the nurse and patient.

Most of the approaches that were confirming used the basic interpersonal techniques set forth by Orlando (1961). These included exploring the patient's perception and definition of the situation (DeVellis, Adams, & DeVellis, 1984; Fuller & Foster, 1982; Powers, Murphy, & Wooldridge, 1983; Powers & Wooldridge, 1982); and use of acknowledgment, reassurance, acceptance, approval, and affirmation (Fuller & Foster, 1982; Salyer & Stuart, 1985).

Drew (1986) described 35 patients' perceptions of confirmation and exclusion behaviors of caregivers. The term *exclusion* evolved from patients' descriptions of their feelings and was defined similarly to disconfirmation. Caregivers who were confirming had an expansive range of affect; were relaxed yet energetic; modulated their voices; avoided jargon; and came close to the patient when speaking. Excluding caregivers were described as having a constricted affect; hurried; disliking their jobs; avoiding eye contact; having a flat tone of voice and abrupt manner of speaking; using jargon or oversimplified language; and avoiding proximity.

Recognition is an essential component of confirmation that is demonstrated by attending to the other. In a study of elderly persons in two chronic care facilities, Rosendahl and Ross (1982) found significant increases in performance on the Goldfarb Mental Status Questionnaire (Kahn, Goldfarb, Polack, & Peck, 1960) when subjects were attended to than when they were not. In this study, attending behavior involved looking at the subject, listening without interruption, and commenting on topics initiated by the subject.

In another study, nursing students' confirming responses were studied. The effects of manipulating types of information given to nurses about the client were investigated to examine the effect on nurses' perception and communication (DeVellis et al., 1984). Fifty-seven nursing students who were given information regarding women's intelligence and decision to remain childless that corresponded to the student's own attitude were found to interact in a more person-centered manner with these clients than with clients who differed from the student. Person-centered responses encouraged clients to disclose what they were experiencing and the meanings these experiences had for them.

Some investigators have sought to determine the effect of confirming communication on the patient by examining patients' physiological changes. Fuller and Foster (1982) examined the effect of family/friend interactions and task-oriented or interpersonally oriented nurse–patient interactions on heart rate, blood pressure, and vocal stress of 28 surgical intensive care unit (SICU) subjects. The interpersonally oriented nurse attempted to draw the patient out, encouraged verbal ventilation, responded to the patient's feelings, sat near the patient, and used touch if warranted. No significant change in cardiovascular variables or vocal stress was found after interactions. Family visits were no more stressful than task or interpersonal nursing visits, and there was no difference between types of nurse visits. These findings were contrasted with the results of other studies using coronary care unit (CCU) patients in which investigators reported a significant increase in heart rate (Brown, 1976; Lynch, Thomas, Mills, & Malinow, 1974). Fuller and Foster (1982) proposed that perhaps SICU patients are less cardiovascularly reactive than CCU patients. This suggestion underscores the importance of replicating studies with different populations of patients.

Deliberative nurse communication that emphasized involving the patient in discussing and working on problems from the patient's point of view was contrasted to a task-oriented approach in attaining social and general health goals in a hypertensive education program (Powers et al., 1983; Powers & Wooldridge, 1982). Reductions in blood pressures of 160 patients were evident with both communication approaches. Although there was a tendency for greater goal attainment in the deliberative group, no significant differences between the approaches were found.

Confirming communication is especially important when the patient is unable to talk. Consequently, the interactions of nurses with 20 intubated intensive care patients were examined using content analysis (Salyer & Stuart, 1985). Positive communication was defined as demonstrating acknowledgment, reassurance, acceptance, approval, or affirmation. Negative communication expressed rejection, refusal, denial, negation, or prohibition. Positive nurse actions most often elicited positive patient reactions, and negative nurse actions most often elicited negative patient reactions. The most frequently observed action–reaction sequence was the nurse action of "silence during administration of patient care" with "no response" from the patient.

In general, despite what patients describe as what they want from interactions with nurses, investigators of confirming communication have not demonstrated conclusively that this type of communication is more effective than disconfirming communication. This result suggests a lack of sensitivity or reliability in instrumentation. In addition, these studies were designed using different labels, operational definitions, and measurement methods. This variability results in difficulty in comparing and contrasting results of studies and in relating the concept of confirmation to other concepts.

In reviewing the section on nurse–patient communication, it is obvious that studies have been conducted in an isolated fashion with no relationship to one another. Despite the importance of communication to the nurse–patient relationship, no research agenda has been identified to provide direction for future research. Kim's model (1987) of the client–nurse domain could provide some direction and offers promise for the future. Kim has suggested that researchers investigate nurse and client characteristics, interaction characteristics, and client outcome criteria.

Despite this lack of a focused direction, some tentative conclusions can be drawn. First, empathic behaviors are not observed consistently by researchers or by patients, and yet patients report a sense of well-being following empathic interventions. There is evidence that patients with different conditions differentially perceive nurse empathy, and there is some support for the conclusion that females are perceived to be more empathic than males.

The studies included in this review provide evidence that regardless of technique, the nurse's intention to focus on the patient resulted in desired outcomes. It is noteworthy that across studies, certain nurse communicative behaviors continue to appear helpful, facilitative, or therapeutic. There is agreement by patients with a variety of diagnoses that the nurse's being available is the most supportive behavior. Both nurses and patients have complained about the availability of nurses, both perhaps aware that being available to one another is essential if nurse–patient communication is to become meaningful.

This research reflects early phases of theoretical development. Investigators have isolated, described, and measured concepts. The concepts of empathy and self-disclosure have been studied longer and have had more precise measurement, as evidenced by the number of instruments designed to measure these phenomena. Most of the studies on empathy and self-disclosure were based on the assumption that these communicative qualities reside in the individual. The implication is that these qualities are independent of the interactive environment. This assumption stands in contrast to the belief that nurse and patient influence one another through their behaviors.

The concepts of support and confirmation are less well described. Description is more difficult, however, because of a belief that these phenomena are interactive. The underlying assumption in confirmation research is that the individual creates meaning through interaction with others in the environment. The individual is not passive but active in shaping the course of events. This assumption calls for complex measurement instruments. The focus is not on measuring individual characteristics but on measuring that which is occurring between or being created by the interaction. Consequently, in these studies the data are the interactions. Methods of data collection generally include nonparticipant observation and audio- or videotaping. Interactions are coded, rated, or classified into categories using rating scales or content analyses. Only a few category systems have been developed and the reliability and validity of these instruments have been assessed and reported incompletely (Garvin, Kennedy, & Cissna, 1988). Not surprisingly, very few category systems have been used in more than one study.

NURSE COMMUNICATIVE ELEMENTS

A variety of nurse characteristics may impact on the nurse's relationship with a client. Nurse communicative elements are the focus of this section.

A few investigators have focused on the effect of type of educational preparation (baccalaureate, diploma, associate degree) on communication characteristics of nurses. Investigators found that type of educational program made a significant difference in nurses' communication abilities (Kunst-Wilson, Carpenter, Poser, Venohr, & Kushner, 1981). This conclusion has confirmed through a meta-analysis conducted by J. H. Johnson (1988).

In other studies of nurse communication characteristics, nurse empathy was the most frequently studied characteristic. Results of the studies were congruent on some findings and conflicting on others. Empathic ability, as measured by the Affective Sensitivity Scale (Schneider, Kagan, & Werner, 1977) and an investigator-developed empathy ability self-report questionnaire, of 66 undergraduate and 50 graduate nursing students compared favorably with the ability of comparably educated individuals in social work, psychology, education, and medicine (Kunst-Wilson et al., 1981). In another study (Williams, 1989) comparing nurse empathy ($n = 143$) with that found in other professions (teaching [$n = 199$] and social work [$n = 50$]), no difference was found by profession; however, women scored significantly higher than men on Mehrabian's Emotional Empathy Scale (Mehrabian & Epstein, 1972) and Stotland's Fantasy-Empathy Scale (Stotland, Mathews, Shermann, Hansson, & Richardson, 1978).

Empathy was not found to be related to nurse age, length of experience (Brunt, 1985; Kunst-Wilson et al., 1981), marital status (Brunt, 1985), or parental status (Brunt, 1985). Brunt (1985) did not find a relationship between empathy and education in 54 nurses from various medical and surgical units. However, Kunst-Wilson et al. (1981) found that the higher educational levels were associated with higher empathy.

In one study (Kunst-Wilson et al., 1981), psychiatric graduate nursing students were found to be more empathic than medical-surgical nursing students when assessed with the Affective Sensitivity Scale (Schneider et al., 1977). In another study (Brunt, 1985), no differences in empathy were found among medical and surgical nurses on the Hogan Empathy Scale (Hogan, 1969), and no relationship was found between technology level on the different units and nurse empathy. These conflicting findings may be a result of the different instruments used to measure empathy or may, in fact, represent actual differences between psychiatric and medical-surgical nurses.

Communication style, as related to education and experience of 150 baccalaureate nursing students, was examined by Harrison, Pistolessi, and Stephen (1989). Using a Q-sort developed by the authors, students described perceptions of their communication behavior. Experience and education were found to affect communication positively and negatively. More advanced students viewed themselves as becoming more sympathetic and egalitarian and less likely to use behaviors that would enhance client responsibility.

Expressiveness versus nonexpressiveness of 173 nurses was examined using responses on an attitude inventory developed to assess attitudes toward patient teaching (Stanton, 1986). Expressiveness was described as interaction that emphasized the setting of mutual goals, whereas nonexpressiveness emphasized a concern with tasks. After classifying items as either expressive or nonexpressive, nurses agreed that a majority of expressive items were more appropriate to patient teaching than nonexpressive items.

In spite of the importance placed on nurses' communication, little sustained research has been conducted on this topic. Demographic variables sometimes were correlated with communication behaviors. The most frequently studied variable was empathy. While many investigators described interactive frameworks to guide their studies, they frequently measured empathy as an individual trait. Nurses were asked to identify feeling states from vignettes or videotapes, but in no case did investigators study actual nurse communication. There is some evidence that self-reported empathy corresponds to the ability to perceive feelings accurately. Nevertheless, the researchers found that nurse empathy was not related to age, marital or parental status, or experience. In addition, baccalaureate education was related positively to desired communication skills in many studies.

PATIENT COMMUNICATIVE ELEMENTS

The other important component in the nurse–patient relationship is the patient. This section reports on patient communicative elements.

In two studies, Hurley (1981, 1983) examined the communication of 68 healthy marital dyads. In both studies, couples were audiotaped in their homes and were asked to resolve their differences on the Inventory of Marital Conflicts (IMC) (Olson & Ryder, 1970), an instrument with vignettes depicting common marital disagreements. Based on the theoretical literature, Hurley hypothesized that pauses, laughter, and interruptions would be related inversely to conflict scores on the IMC and inversely to the amount of stress during the conflict-stimulated interaction. The above-mentioned communication behaviors were believed to be indicative of spontaneity and flexibility in the family system and, therefore, were expected to be present in the interaction of nonconflicted, nonstressed couples. The hypotheses were not supported in either study, and, in part, the findings were attributed to the simulated laboratory situation. Of interest, however, was that the communication variables were intercorrelated, suggesting a style of communication that could be used in family system assessment.

Baer and Lowery (1987) examined patient characteristics that influenced the feelings of 140 baccalaureate nursing students. Students liked best caring for persons who were male, tidy, ambulatory, cheerful, and communicative. They liked caring for patients who showed some appreciation for the help they were trying to give. The findings of this study highlight the fact that patient communication characteristics are important variables to consider when examining the nurse–patient relationship.

In a comparison of the communication characteristics of four psychiatric patient groups and a group of nursing students, Heineken (1982) found that three out of the four psychiatric groups had higher disconfirmation frequencies than the student group. Disconfirmation generally was defined as dysfunctional communicative behavior. The findings were consistent with what one would expect from the theory and suggested a way that mentally ill persons might contribute to their known difficulty in establishing and maintaining relationships.

In a study of a specific dysfunctional communication behavior, Topf (1988) examined interpersonal responsiveness of 33 male Veterans Administration psychiatric patients. The investigator reported that the degree of patient expressiveness was correlated positively with (a) the average number of words spoken, (b) the average number of feelings expressed, (c) the percentage of one-word speech utterances, and (d) the average level of intimacy for speech utterances. Topf used these findings to develop an instrument for nurses to assess patient interpersonal responsiveness. Methods of intervention also were suggested.

In a test of the effect of engagement on blood pressure, Smyth, Sparacino, Hansell, and Call (1980) asked 31 black inner-city women to converse informally with a nurse while their blood pressures were monitored. Engagement was a broad term used to refer to the degree of involvement in an interaction. Type A and hypertensive subjects were judged not to display greater engagement than type B and normotensive subjects, respectively. One component of engagement involves the contemplation and revelation of personal information (self-disclosure). Although the investigators found no significant relationship between engagement and increased blood pressure, they cautioned nurses to be alert to the likelihood that intense emotions may distort blood pressure and other critical measurements.

Another study was focused on patient physiological responses during communication with nurses. During nurse interaction with 19 coronary care patients, two major cardiovascular changes were observed (Thomas et al., 1982). Most of the patients had a significant increase in heart rate during interaction compared with preinteraction rates. Second, postinteraction heart rates were significantly lower than preinteraction heart rates. The investigators noted, however, the unique cardiovascular response of each patient.

Smith and Cantrell (1988) designed an experiment in which physical and verbal aspects of personal space served as the independent variables in a study on patient anxiety and heart rate. One registered nurse varied her physical distance and type of questions (personal or impersonal) while individually interacting with 40 inpatient VA schizophrenic patients. The investigators found no differences in anxiety, but patient heart rate was increased significantly when the nurse asked personal questions, regardless of distance from the patient. The investigators suggested that the verbal impact of nurses may be negative if nurses are overly intrusive in their verbal interactions with patients.

In another study on the relationship between cardiovascular variables and communication characteristics, 48 hypertensive patients' diastolic blood pressures were found to be significantly higher during reading aloud than when sitting quietly (Hellman & Grimm, 1984). These findings indicate that patients show significant cardiovascular responses when talking.

Although not large in number, the studies on communication characteristics of patients provide interesting findings that should influence practice. What little research has been done on patient communicative elements has been diverse in terms of subject selection. Studies have been focused on the full range of the health continuum, including healthy couples in their homes, outpatients, and patients in intensive care. Investigators who have studied patients with a variety of diagnoses have suggested that there are differences in the ways patients perceive others' communications and in the way they communicate.

No instrument was used in more than one study. Several instruments were investigator-designed, with only minimal information reported on psychometric properties. Recent studies provide evidence that investigators are making serious efforts to use and/or develop reliable and valid instruments.

All but two of the studies on patient communicative elements were descriptive in nature, with three correlating communication with other variables or other communicative behaviors. Unlike the studies on nurse characteristics, investigators more consistently collected naturally occurring communication data on patient–nurse interactions. Most data were collected on audiotapes.

The work to date on patient characteristics provides some scientific documentation of actual communication behavior. Some of the research confirms one's intuitive sense, for example, that psychiatric patients are not interpersonally responsive. Other results are unexpected, for example, that pulse rate increased with personal questions and while talking. Without this documentation, nurses have only their hunches and experience on which to base care. Much more documentation of behavior is needed.

SUGGESTIONS FOR FUTURE RESEARCH

Future research based on frameworks that are clear about the interactive nature of nurse–patient communication should be designed to describe the process, content, and outcomes of nurse–patient interactions (Lynn, 1987). It is important that investigators critically analyze and build on the work of others in developing their conceptual and operational definitions of the concepts under study.

Process, content, and outcomes also should be examined as they change according to the phases of the nurse–patient relationship. What communication behaviors are actually employed by nurses in the orientation, working, and resolution phases? What communication behaviors are most effective in creating positive patient outcomes in each phase of the relationship? Further, what are the implications of timing under the current conditions of brief hospitalization and short-term relationships?

All types of nurse–patient interactions should be the focus of systematic study. Research on communication behaviors as they are affected by age, race, gender, and culture of both interactants is needed. In addition, how does the diagnosis of the patient affect the communication? For example, M. N. Johnson (1980) suggested that the communication behaviors that are appropriate in the medical-surgical area may be different from those that would be most effective with psychiatric patients. The problems associated with convenience samples need to be overcome by careful attention to design in order to answer these research questions.

One of the most pressing needs is for better instrumentation. Instruments that are congruent with the theoretical frameworks need to be developed and used in more than one program of research. Another issue relates to the perspective from which the concepts are measured. Certainly the patient's perception of communication qualities is paramount in the nursing process. In addition, there are observable strategies common among nurses' approaches to patients in certain situations that can be named, described, and explained. Instruments that can measure these behavioral qualities sensitively are needed. Physiological measures may be more sensitive to changes in patient condition than some of the psychosocial measures, and thus the significance of intervention may be more readily ascertained (Smith & Cantrell, 1988). Triangulation in measurement with the goal of congruence among self-report, observed, and physiological measures of outcome is an important future direction.

Methods of data collection that record the actual communication of the nurse and patient, such as audio- and videotape recordings, are needed to gather reliable and valid data. Actual communication versus measures of contemplated or self-reported communication increasingly must serve as a valid source of data. Methods that involve the collection of actual communication, however, are expensive, time-consuming, and sometimes intrusive. It is important that researchers take advantage of the advancing technologies, such as telemetry, to correlate physiological variables with communication variables. Use of information stored in computer memory banks increasingly can be used for research.

As the types of data change from individual data to interactive data, the assumption of independence necessary for many of the current statistical tests will not be met. Data analysis techniques necessarily will change as the types of research questions and data collection techniques change. Procedures such as time-series analysis increasingly will be necessary to describe interactional processes, content, and outcomes. Further development of communication rating scales will involve the use of category systems. Much work needs to be done to develop valid and reliable category systems.

Other fruitful approaches to data analysis include discourse analysis and ethnographic analysis. These approaches take into account the situated nature of communication, that is, that communication takes place in specific contexts that must be made explicit in order to understand the communication. Both of these approaches allow examination of actual nurse–patient communication. Discourse analysis is a microanalysis of the structure and pragmatics of the interaction. Ethnographic analysis involves larger units of interaction data. Use of both approaches will help to identify and describe the essential concepts necessary for understanding nurse–patient communication.

The findings of the studies reported in this review are a beginning attempt to define important communication concepts necessary in effective nurse–patient communication. It is evident that the first level of theory development, that of factor-naming (Dickoff & James, 1968), has not been achieved entirely. Progress in factor-relating, predictive, or prescriptive theory rests on the adequacy with which communication concepts are named, described, and measured. Further research is needed to develop a systematic body of knowledge to guide effective communication in nursing practice.

REFERENCES

Baer, E. D., & Lowery, B. J. (1987). Patient and situational factors that affect nursing students' like or dislike of caring for patients. *Nursing Research, 36,* 298–302.

Bales, R. F. (1950). *Interaction process analysis: A method for the study of small groups.* Cambridge, MA: Addison-Wesley.

Brown, A. J. (1976). Effect of family visits on the blood pressure and heart rate of patients in the coronary care unit. *Heart & Lung, 5,* 291–296.

Brunt, J. H. (1985). An exploration of the relationship between nurses' empathy and technology. *Nursing Administration Quarterly, 9*(4), 69–78.

Chinn, P. L., & Jacobs, M. K. (1987). *Theory and nursing.* St. Louis, MO: Mosby.

Dawson, C. (1985). Hypertension, perceived clinician empathy and patient self-disclosure. *Research in Nursing & Health, 8,* 191–198.

DeVellis, B. M., Adams, J. L., & DeVellis, R. F. (1984). Effects of information on patient stereotyping. *Research in Nursing & Health, 7,* 237–244.

Dickoff, G., & James, P. A. (1968). A theory of theories: A position paper. *Nursing Research, 17,* 197–203.

Diers, D., & Leonard, R. C. (1966). Interaction analysis in nursing research. *Nursing Research, 15,* 225–228.

Drew, N. (1986). Exclusion and confirmation: A phenomenology of patients' experiences with care givers. *Image: Journal of Nursing Scholarship, 18,* 39–43.

Fuller, B. F., & Foster, G. M. (1982). The effects of family/friend visits vs. staff interaction on stress/arousal of surgical intensive care patients. *Heart & Lung, 11,* 457–463.

Gardner, K. G., & Wheeler, E. C. (1987). Patients' perceptions of support. *Western Journal of Nursing Research, 9,* 115–131.

Garvin, B. J., Kennedy, C. W., & Cissna, K. N. (1988). Reliability in category coding systems. *Nursing Research, 37*, 52–55.

Gurman, A. S. (1977). The patient's perception of therapeutic relationship. In A. S. Gurman & A. M. Razin (Eds.), *Effective psychotherapy: A handbook of research* (pp. 503–543). New York: Pergamon.

Harrison, T. M., Pistolessi, T. V., & Stephen, T. D. (1989). Assessing nurses' communication: A cross-sectional study. *Western Journal of Nursing Research, 11*, 75–91.

Heineken, J. (1982). Disconfirmation in dysfunctional communication. *Nursing Research, 31*, 211–213.

Hellman, R., & Grimm, S. A. (1984). The influence of talking on diastolic blood pressure readings. *Research in Nursing & Health, 7*, 253–256.

Hogan, R. (1969). Development of an empathy scale. *Journal of Consulting and Clinical Psychology, 33*, 307–316.

Hurley, P. M. (1981). Communication patterns and conflict in marital dyads. *Nursing Research, 30*, 38–42.

Hurley, P. M. (1983). Communication variables and voice analysis of marital conflict stress. *Nursing Research, 32*, 164–169.

Johnson, J. H. (1988). Differences in the performances of baccalaureate, associate degree, and diploma nurses: A meta-analysis. *Research in Nursing & Health, 11*, 183–197.

Johnson, M. N. (1980). Self-disclosure: A variable in the nurse–client relationship. *Journal of Psychiatric Nursing and Mental Health Services, 18*(1), 17–20.

Jourard, S. M. (1971). *The transparent self.* New York: Van Nostrand Reinhold.

Kahn, R., Goldfarb, A., Polack, M., & Peck, A. (1960). Brief objective measures for the determination of mental status in the aged. *American Journal of Psychiatry, 117*, 326–328.

Kim, H. S. (1987). Structuring the nursing knowledge system: A typology of four domains. *Scholarly Inquiry for Nursing Practice, 1*, 99–114.

Kishi, K. I. (1983). Communication patterns of health teaching and information recall. *Nursing Research, 32*, 230–235.

Kunst-Wilson, W., Carpenter, L., Poser, A., Venohr, I., & Kushner, K. (1981). Empathic perceptions of nursing students: Self-reported and actual ability. *Research in Nursing & Health, 4*, 283–293.

Laing, R. D. (1969). *The self and others.* Baltimore, MD: Penguin.

La Monica, E. (1981). Construct validity of an empathy instrument. *Research in Nursing & Health, 4*, 389–400.

La Monica, E. L., Wolf, R. M., Madea, A. R., & Oberst, M. T. (1987). Empathy and nursing outcomes. *Scholarly Inquiry for Nursing Practice, 1*, 197–213.

Limandri, B. J. (1987). The therapeutic relationship with abused women. *Journal of Psychosocial Nursing and Mental Health Services, 25*(2), 9–16.

Lynch, J. J., Thomas, S. A., Mills, M. E., & Malinow, K. (1974). The effects of human contact on cardiac arrhythmia in coronary care patients. *Journal of Nervous and Mental Disease, 158*, 88–89.

Lynn, M. R. (1987). Pediatric nurse practitioner–patient interactions: A study of the process. *Journal of Pediatric Nursing, 2*, 268–271.

Mehrabian, A., & Epstein, N. (1972). A measure of emotional empathy. *Journal of Personality, 40*, 525–543.

Morgan, B. S., & Barden, M. E. (1985). Nurse–patient interaction in the home setting. *Public Health Nursing, 2,* 159–167.

Niemeier, D. F. (1983). A behavioral analysis of staff–patient interactions in a psychiatric setting. *Western Journal of Nursing Research, 5,* 269–277.

Northouse, P. G., & Northouse, L. L. (1985). *Health communication.* Englewood Cliffs, NJ: Prentice-Hall.

Olson, D. H., & Ryder, R. G. (1970). Inventory of Marital Conflicts (IMC): An experimental interaction procedure. *Journal of Marriage and the Family, 32,* 443–448.

Orlando, I. J. (1961). *The dynamic nurse–patient relationship.* New York: Putnam.

Peplau, H. (1975). Talking with patients. In A. Marrimer (Ed.), *The nursing process: A scientific approach to nursing care* (pp. 161–165). St. Louis, MO: Mosby.

Powers, M. J., Murphy, S. P., & Wooldridge, P. J. (1983). Validation of two experimental nursing approaches using content analysis. *Research in Nursing & Health, 6,* 3–9.

Powers, M. J., & Wooldridge, P. J. (1982). Factors influencing knowledge, attitudes and compliance of hypertensive patients. *Research in Nursing & Health, 5,* 171–182.

Rogers, C. R. (1975). Empathic: An unappreciated way of being. *The Counseling Psychologist, 5*(2), 2–10.

Rosendahl, P. P., & Ross, V. (1982). Does your behavior affect your patient's response? *Journal of Gerontological Nursing, 8,* 572–575.

Salyer, J., & Stuart, B. J. (1985). Nurse–patient interaction in the intensive care unit. *Heart & Lung, 14,* 20–24.

Schneider, J., Kagan, N., & Werner, D. (1977, August). *The development of a measure of empathy: The Affective Empathy Scale.* Paper presented at the 85th meeting of the American Psychological Association, San Francisco.

Simon, S., Wilson, B., & Munjas, B. A. (1982). Are nursing personnel reinforcing mental illness? *Virginia Nurse, 50*(4), 55–57.

Slavinsky, A. T., & Krauss, J. B. (1982). Two approaches to the management of long-term psychiatric outpatients in the community. *Nursing Research, 31,* 284–289.

Smith, B. J., & Cantrell, P. J. (1988). Distance in nurse–patient encounters. *Journal of Psychosocial Nursing and Mental Health Services, 26*(2), 22–26.

Smyth, K., Sparacino, J., Hansell, S., & Call, J. (1980). Engagement–involvement and blood pressure change: A methodological inquiry. *Nursing Research, 29,* 270–275.

Stanton, M. P. (1986). Nurses' attitudes toward nurse–patient interaction in the patient-teaching situation. *Nursing Success Today, 3*(4), 12–19.

Stotland, E., Mathews, K. E., Sherman, S. E., Hansson, R. O., & Richardson, B. A. (1978). *Empathy, fantasy, and helping.* Beverly Hills, CA: Sage.

Thomas, S. A., Friedmann, E., Noctor, M., Sappington, E., Gross, H., & Lynch, J. J. (1982). Patients' cardiac responses to nursing interviews in a CCU. *Dimensions of Critical Care, 1,* 198–205.

Topf, M. (1988). Verbal interpersonal responsibilities. *Journal of Psychosocial Nursing and Mental Health Services, 26*(7), 8–16.

Trandel-Korenchuk, D. M. (1987). The effect of social and care environments on the disclosure practices of nurse midwives relative to methods of pain management in childbirth. *Journal of Obstetric, Gynecologic, and Neonatal Nursing, 16,* 258–265.

Webster-Stratton, C. (1984). *PNP interpersonal behavior constructs: A means for analyzing videotaped dyadic interaction. A manual.* Unpublished manuscript.

Webster-Stratton, C., Glascock, J., & McCarthy, A. M. (1986). Nurse practitioner–patient interactional analyses during well-child visits. *Nursing Research, 35,* 247–249.

Weiss, S. J. (1988). Touch. In J. J. Fitzpatrick, R. L. Taunton, & J. Q. Beneliel (Eds.), *Annual Review of Nursing Research* (pp. 3–27). New York: Springer Publishing.

Williams, C. A. (1989). Empathy and burnout in male and female helping professionals. *Research in Nursing & Health, 12,* 169–178.

Young, J. C. (1988). Rationale for clinical self-disclosure and research agenda. *Image: Journal of Nursing Scholarship, 20,* 196–199.

Index

Contents of Previous Volumes

VOLUME V

ORDER FORM

Save 10% on Volume 9 with this coupon.

__ Check here to order the ANNUAL REVIEW OF NURSING RESEARCH, Volume 9, 1991 at a 10% discount. You will receive an invoice requesting pre-payment.

Save 10% on all future volumes with a continuation order.

__ Check here to place your continuation order for the ANNUAL REVIEW OF NURSING RESEARCH. You will receive a pre-payment invoice with a 10% discount upon publication of each new volume, beginning with Volume 9, 1991. You may pay for prompt shipment or cancel with no obligation.

Name _____

Institution _____

Address _____

City/State/Zip _____

Examination copies for possible course adoption are available to instructors "on approval" only. Write on institutional letterhead, noting course, level, present text, and expected enrollment (Include $2.50 for postage and handling). Prices slightly higher overseas. Prices subject to change.

Mail this coupon to:
SPRINGER PUBLISHING COMPANY
536 Broadway, New York, N.Y. 10012